ABC of
Colorectal Cancer

Second Edition

ABC series

An outstanding collection of resources – written by specialists for non-specialists

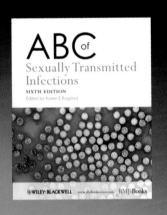

ABC of Sexually Transmitted Infections
SIXTH EDITION
Edited by Karen E Rogstad

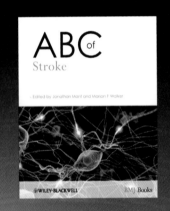

ABC of Stroke
Edited by Jonathan Mant and Marion F. Walker

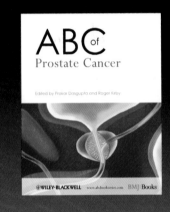

ABC of Prostate Cancer
Edited by Prokar Dasgupta and Roger Kirby

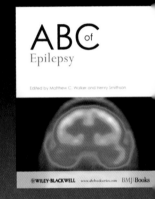

ABC of Epilepsy
Edited by Matthew C. Walker and Henry Smithson

The *ABC* series contains a wealth of indispensable resources for GPs, GP registrars, junior doctors, doctors in training and all those in primary care

▶ **Now fully revised and updated**

▶ **Highly illustrated, informative and a practical source of knowledge**

▶ **An easy-to-use resource, covering the symptoms, investigations, treatment and management of conditions presenting in day-to-day practice and patient support**

▶ **Full colour photographs and illustrations aid diagnosis and patient understanding of a condition**

For more information on all books in the *ABC* series, including links to further information, references and links to the latest official guidelines, please visit:

www.abcbookseries.com

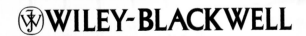

BMJ|Books

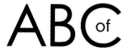

ABC of

Colorectal Cancer

Second Edition

EDITED BY

Annie Young

Professor of Nursing, Warwick Medical School
The University of Warwick, Coventry, UK

Richard Hobbs

Professor and Head of Primary Care Health Sciences
Department of Primary Care Health Sciences
University of Oxford, Oxford, UK

David Kerr

Professor of Cancer Medicine
Nuffield Department of Clinical and Laboratory Sciences
University of Oxford, Oxford, UK

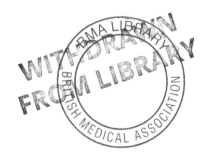
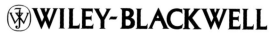

WILEY-BLACKWELL

A John Wiley & Sons, Ltd., Publication

BMJ|Books

This edition first published 2011, © 2011 by Blackwell Publishing Ltd

BMJ Books is an imprint of BMJ Publishing Group Limited, used under licence by Blackwell Publishing which was acquired by John Wiley & Sons in February 2007. Blackwell's publishing programme has been merged with Wiley's global Scientific, Technical and Medical business to form Wiley-Blackwell.

Registered office: John Wiley & Sons, Ltd, The Atrium, Southern Gate, Chichester, West Sussex, PO19 8SQ, UK

Editorial offices: 9600 Garsington Road, Oxford, OX4 2DQ, UK
The Atrium, Southern Gate, Chichester, West Sussex, PO19 8SQ, UK
111 River Street, Hoboken, NJ 07030-5774, USA

For details of our global editorial offices, for customer services and for information about how to apply for permission to reuse the copyright material in this book please see our website at www.wiley.com/wiley-blackwell

Library of Congress Cataloging-in-Publication Data
ABC of colorectal cancer / edited by Annie Young, Richard Hobbs, David Kerr. – 2nd ed.
    p. ; cm.
  Includes bibliographical references and index.
  ISBN-13: 978-1-4051-7763-4 (pbk. : alk. paper)
  ISBN-10: 1-4051-7763-2
  1. Colon (Anatomy) – Cancer – Treatment. 2. Rectum – Cancer – Treatment. I. Young, Annie M. (Annie Miller), 1955-
II. Hobbs, Richard, M.R.C.G.P. III. Kerr, David J.
  [DNLM: 1. Colorectal Neoplasms. WI 529]
  RC280.C6A23 2011
  616.99′4347 – dc23
                                                                                         2011013471

A catalogue record for this book is available from the British Library.
This book is published in the following electronic formats: ePDF 9781444346435; ePub 9781444346442; Mobi 9781444346459

Set in 9.25/12 Minion by Laserwords Private Limited, Chennai, India
Printed and bound in Malaysia by Vivar Printing Sdn Bhd

1 2011

Contents

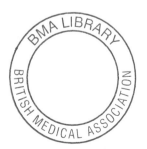

Contributors

Shazad Ashraf
Specialist Registrar in Colorectal Surgery
Department of Colorectal Surgery, John Radcliffe Hospital,
Oxford, UK

Wendy S Atkin
Professor of Gastrointestinal Epidemiology
Imperial College London, London, UK

Mark Austin
Senior Software Developer
IXICO Ltd, London, UK

Kevin Bond
Cancer Patient, Worcester, UK

Vicky Bowyer
Research Fellow
Health Sciences Research Institute, Warwick Medical School,
The University of Warwick, Coventry, UK

Peter Boyle
Professor of Epidemiology and Prevention
International Prevention Research Institute, Lyon,
France

Joanne L Brady
Clinical Research Fellow
Department of Oncology, Churchill Hospital, Oxford, UK

Sir Michael Brady
Department of Radiation Oncology and Biology
Old Road Campus Research Building, Oxford, UK

Michael Christie
Consultant Anatomical Pathologist
Royal Melbourne Hospital, Melbourne, Australia

Trevor Cole
Consultant in Clinical and Cancer Genetics
Birmingham Women's NHS Foundation Trust,
Birmingham, UK

David Cunningham
Head of GI/Lymphoma Unit
Department of Medicine, The Royal Marsden
NHS Foundation Trust, Royal Marsden Hospital, London and Surrey, UK

Maria Paula Curado
Professor of Epidemiology and Prevention
International Prevention Research Institute, Lyon, France

Richard Hobbs
Professor and Head of Primary Care Health Sciences
Department of Primary Care Health Sciences,
University of Oxford, Oxford, UK

Mohammad Ilyas
Professor of Pathology
University of Nottingham, Queen's Medical Centre, Nottingham, UK

Matthew Kelly
Senior Scientist
Siemens Molecular Imaging, Oxford, UK

David Kerr
Professor of Cancer Medicine
Nuffield Departement of Clinical and Laboratory Sciences,
University of Oxford, Oxford, UK

Pauline McCulloch
Community Palliaitve Care CNS
North West Central london PCt, Camden Provider Services
Islington Palliaitve Care Service, London, UK

Neil Mortensen
Professor of Colorectal Surgery
Department of Colorectal Surgery, John Radcliffe Hospital, Oxford, UK

Patrick Mullie
Professor of Epidemiology and Prevention
International Prevention Research Institute, Lyon, France

Kai Ren Ong
Consultant in Clinical and Cancer Genetics
Birmingham Women's NHS Foundation Trust, Birmingham, UK

Julietta Patnick

Director, NHS Cancer Screening Programmes
Visiting Professor, Oxford University, UK

John Primrose

Professor of Surgery
Southampton General Hospital, Southampton, UK

Zenia Saridaki-Zoras

Medical Oncologist Research Fellow
Laboratory of Tumor Cell Biology, Medical School, University of Crete, Crete, Greece

Oliver Sieber

Joint Laboratory Head
Ludwig Colon Cancer Initiative Laboratory,
Ludwig Institute for Cancer Research, Parkville, Australia

Andrew Slater

Consultant Radiologist
John Radcliffe Hospital, Oxford, UK

David Watkins

Research Fellow
Department of Medicine, The Royal Marsden NHS Foundation Trust,
Royal Marsden Hospital, London and Surrey, UK

Andrew Weaver

Department of Oncology, Churchill Hospital, Oxford, UK

Sue Wilson

Professor of Clinical Epidemiology
University of Birmingham, Birmingham, UK

Annie Young

Professor of Nursing
Warwick Medical School, The University of Warwick,
Coventry, UK

David Zaridze

Institute of Carcinogenesis, Moscow, Russian Federation

Preface

Colorectal cancer is a common source of morbidity and mortality, with an estimated 1 million incident cases every year, predominantly in Western nations. The truism, 'biology is king' is especially applicable to colorectal cancer as we have come to understand the epidemiological interplay between genetics and the environment, the molecular biology of the progression from benign adenoma to invasive carcinoma and the biomarkers which identify which patients might benefit most from specific therapies. It is a cancer which lends itself to prevention, screening and early detection and which cries out for a multidisciplinary approach, underpinned by the innovative IT and decision support described in Chapter 6. Optimal management extends from population screening, through primary care to secondary and specialist tertiary centres, encapsulating the microcosm of modern cancer care.

We provide updates on important advances in genetics, screening and treatment and include a moving chapter written by a patient who captures the highs and lows, the small indignities and the great kindnesses of his own cancer pathway. We cover the entire spectrum of the disease in a lucid style with an outstanding faculty, each of whom has the capacity for the clarity of communication required to bring the reader up to date with the latest advances which make a real difference to the clinical management of this disease.

You will read, enjoy and reread this book if you are a GP in the front line of cancer care; if you are a medical student who wants to understand the essence of multidisciplinary cancer diagnosis and treatment; if you are a nurse specialist who wants to develop the knowledge base to support your patients at every step of their care pathway; if you are a medical or surgical trainee interested in the management of colorectal cancer.

Remember the patient's (and the endoscopist's!) battle-cry, 'E Tenebris Lux'.

Annie Young
Richard Hobbs
David Kerr

CHAPTER 1

The Patient Perspective

Kevin Bond

Cancer patient, Worcester, UK

OVERVIEW

- The family environment and the support it offers hugely influence how the patient deals with a diagnosis of colorectal cancer
- Surveys suggest that colorectal cancer patients seem generally grateful and satisfied with their treatment, including the quality and timeliness of the information they received, the quality of their healthcare, and their level of involvement in decision making
- Nevertheless, despite progress, individual coordination of care still needs addressing, particularly around long-term follow up
- Patients generally have a relatively positive outlook on their illness experience, although those with colostomies have some added difficulty and side effects of treatment often cause anxiety
- Patients need the whole team approach to manage overall care, and to act as a sounding board for ideas and treatment options – not only family and friends and cancer specialists, but GPs and allied healthcare professionals
- Clarity of communication, based on honesty and openness, is key

Coping with ill-health: family influences

Our views are not shaped through our isolated experience of life alone but also through our upbringing and family influences. The metaphysical poet John Donne said, 'no man is an island unto himself'. I therefore feel that it is appropriate to mention relative family influences which have obviously impacted on how I view the experience of dealing with colorectal cancer. This could be considered a different angle on personalised medicine, in which genetics are trumped by nurture.

My parents came to England from Ireland in the 1930s. My father was a maintenance electrician in a large machine tool manufacturer and my mother was a nursing Sister having qualified in both mental and general nursing. My mother's sister also became a nurse. My

ABC of Colorectal Cancer, Second Edition.
Edited by Annie Young, Richard Hobbs and David Kerr.
© 2011 Blackwell Publishing Ltd. Published 2011 by Blackwell Publishing Ltd.

paternal grandmother was a midwife, as was my father's sister. I learned of the many advances made in medicine over their careers but also of its limitations and the gentle grace with which this was accepted.

My wife has specialised in elderly care and neuro-physiotherapy and for the past five years has been the physiotherapist at St Richards Hospice, Worcester. This makes life for her at the moment more rather than less difficult; she is more than well acquainted with the prognosis of my illness. Ignorance can sometimes have its blessings, if only in the short term.

Attitude matters!

I am an Incorporated Engineer and have been a director within several companies since 1976. The one thing I have found is that there is usually more than one view or resolution to any complex problem and there is normally a safe default attitude, bowing to the view of a glass being half empty. My gift lay with a logical appreciation of the technical argument, exploring and exposing possible alternatives and moving the argument and solution to one of a glass half full and getting more full! It is rare to find only one solution and for that solution to be perfect, without ongoing or unforeseen problems that have to be managed or mitigated. Therefore my expectations in expressing a patient's view are conditioned with a sense of reality. I am aware that NHS funds are not limitless and that there are others much worse off than me. This does not, however, stop me from exploring that which is or might still be possible and using every scrap of available information to empower this journey.

Signs and symptoms: get medical help as soon as possible

The first real noticeable symptoms of my illness manifested themselves in early 2007 and the regularity and severity of these increased as the year progressed. These included:

- increased flatulence
- feeling bloated
- feeling abdominal discomfort within an hour or so of eating
- having to repeatedly go to the toilet

- blood staining on toilet paper
- actually passing blood with stools
- having to go to the toilet during the night.

At first I was not too concerned as I had irritable bowel syndrome from time to time and had piles, and so to begin with had thought it was just a combination of these two. As the year progressed, my wife became more concerned and badgered me to see my GP but, typical of the male species, I put the matter off; after all, on occasions the symptoms would ease and almost disappear. Besides I had always been very fit and healthy (sporting injuries apart). I was never ill and hardly knew my way to the GP's surgery. Also, I was now in business with another colleague and I could not afford the time to be ill! My wife settled the matter and told me she had made an appointment for me with our GP (I had had the symptoms for 12 months by then) and my subsequent history can be summarised as follows:

- Late November 2007 – Initial consultation at GP surgery.
- Early December 2007 – Blood test appointment.
- January 2008 – Endoscopy appointment with consultant surgeon at Worcestershire Royal at which she informed me there were tumours and they were, from her experience unlikely to be benign. Appointments followed for MRI and CT scans.
- February 2008 – Consultation with surgeon to review results of scans which indicated the colon tumour had metastasised to the liver, then colon resection and referral to the liver unit in Birmingham for possible liver resection
- May to July 2008 – Referred to Cheltenham General Hospital for chemotherapy regime of six fortnightly sessions of Oxaliplatin and 5-Fluorouracil (5-FU)
- 2009 – Liver resection at St James's Hospital, Leeds
- 2010 – One further course of chemotherapy locally at Worcestershire Royal Hospital.

Good communication throughout the care pathway is the golden key

So breaking bad news was done sensitively and in stages – after the endoscopy and scans with my wife present at each consultation. Although a massive shock, I was grateful for the frankness at each stage which meant there was no false expectation at any of the appointments, which had been in quick succession. I heard 'cancer' and 'secondaries' and little else and was grateful for my wife's attendance and the written, explanatory notes which we could take home to study.

Good to have a plan of action

I appreciated a plan of action to focus my mind. I became involved – saw the stoma nurse as a colostomy was a possibility at the time of surgery; saw a liver surgeon – to keep that in reserve for after chemotherapy. After my bowel resection (and thankfully, I didn't need a colostomy), I set about self-made plan to get fit for chemotherapy – to eat healthy food, to exercise avidly and to show patience and endurance throughout adversity.

Telling my sons, mother and three brothers

The worst bit about the diagnosis and pathway was telling my sons, mother and three brothers. As an ex-nurse, my mum was able to be rational and positive. I had to ask my elder son to come back from Iceland early and summon my younger son, who had just started university in Wales, to come home. We had never talked about cancer ever as a family but my son immediately told me that a friend of his had been diagnosed with testicular cancer, which made my problem seem small in comparison.

Rationalising having cancer

I didn't do the 'Why me?' question that fellow patients speak of, as that seems unresolvable and a waste of my energies. I had had a good life, travelled over the world and been fortunate to raise a lovely family – so felt fortunate. Emotionally, it's tough. I still contemplate all things that I thought I'd do, my dreams and expectations that, for various reasons, are out of reach now; we can no longer afford some of them, my earning capacity has been curtailed as I owned my own business. I have a different focus now, sadly taken up with treatment regimes ahead of me, and am unlikely to be fit enough to realise most of my dreams. So I keep it simple – what else is there other than a return to as reasonable a life as possible within one's own family?

As much as possible, I carry on with work; the stark reality is that the mortgage has to be paid, but we do need more information on what benefits the State might provide.

My colorectal cancer pathway

Due to the pattern of the care, my cancer pathway has had highs and lows, moments of high drama, low humour, encouragement and disappointment. As I write I find that, despite the best treatment that the NHS could offer and the indefatigable support of my wife and family, the cancer has recurred yet again and that there is no prospect now of cure. In some ways I am glad to be spared further chemotherapy at the moment, as the last session proved tough. My focus now is on keeping as fit and comfortable as possible, supported as I have been throughout by those constant companions, my family and GP. I know that I can access supportive and palliative care services if required, having already been introduced to my palliative care nurse.

I know that I have lived longer than if I had been diagnosed 10 years ago and that I may soon exhaust conventional medical approaches. I may consider complementary therapies but will avoid procedures that might make me feel worse.

Don't believe everything you read on the internet, but feel free to take control of your own life and travel hopefully. This I intend to do.

Acknowledgement

At a time when criticism of the National Health Service (NHS) still remains politically convenient, I can only report that once I was actively placed with the appropriate consultant, the care I received for the three and a half years since November 2007 of my illness was generally first class. For the greater part, it would be hard to imagine that even the most expensive of private health care could offer very much more.

I do refer to certain criticisms of the NHS, but I would not want to appear to be churlish or ungrateful – far from it. The criticisms are to be constructive and serve to help others.

May I express my deepest gratitude to all the staff within Worcestershire Royal Hospital, Cheltenham General Hospital, St James' Hospital, Leeds and Queen Elizabeth Hospital, Birmingham, as well as my General Practitioner, Knightwick Surgery, Worcestershire and the Community Nurses for their professional skill and the kindness they have shown me.

Further reading

Useful websites for both patients and professionals:

American Cancer Society http://www.cancer.org/docroot/MLT/content/MLT _4_1x_Living_With_Uncertainty_-_The_Fear_of_Cancer_Recurrence.asp [accessed 10 April 2011].

Beating Bowel Cancer http://www.beatingbowelcancer.org/ [accessed 10 April 2011].

Bowel Cancer UK http://www.bowelcanceruk.org.uk [accessed 10 April 2011].

The Lance Armstrong Foundation http://www.livestrong.org/site/ c.khLXK1PxHmF/b.2660683/k.5BD8/Sadness_and_Depression.htm [accessed 10 April 2010].

MacmillanCancerBackup http://www.macmillan.org.uk/Cancerinformation/ Livingwithandaftercancer/Relationshipscommunication/Sexuality/ Solutionstosexualproblems.aspx [accessed 10 April 2010].

CHAPTER 2

Epidemiology and Prevention

Peter Boyle[1], *Patrick Mullie*[1], *Maria Paula Curado*[1] *and David Zaridze*[2]

[1]International Prevention Research Institute, Lyon, France
[2]Institute of Carcinogenesis, Moscow, Russian Federation

OVERVIEW

The most important lifestyle changes for colorectal cancer disease prevention are as follows:

- Stop smoking
- Reduce alcohol consumption
- Increase physical activity
- Adopt a healthier diet: low in red/processed meats, high in fruit, vegetables, whole grains and dietary fibre

Further research on gene–diet interactions and identifying protective dietary and lifestyle patterns is required

---

Introduction

Colorectal cancer is an important public health problem throughout the world. It is the third most common cancer in men (663,000 cases in 2008: 10% of all cancer cases) and the second in women (570,000 cases: 9.4% of all cancer cases) worldwide. Significant international variations in the distribution of colorectal cancer have been observed for many years. High incidence rates are found in Western Europe and North America, intermediate rates in Eastern Europe with the lowest rates to be found in sub-Saharan Africa (Figure 2.1).

About 608,000 deaths from colorectal cancer are estimated worldwide, accounting for 8% of all cancer deaths, making it the fourth most common cause of death from cancer. As observed for incidence, mortality rates are lower in women than in men; with less variability in mortality rates worldwide (sixfold in men (Figure 2.2) and fivefold in women). Like most solid tumours, the incidence of colorectal cancer increases with age (with the exception of familial colorectal cancer) and, in most regions of the world, the incidence of colorectal cancer is increasing and the mortality rate decreasing (Figures 2.3 and 2.4). The incidence of colon cancer is uniformly higher than rectal cancer in both men and women.

Aetiology of colorectal cancer

Ethnic and racial differences in colorectal cancer incidence as well as studies on migrants have suggested for many years that environmental factors play a major role for the aetiology of the disease. In Israel, male Jews born in Europe or America were shown to be at higher risk for colon cancer than those born in Africa or Asia, and a change in risk in the offspring of Japanese having migrated to the United States has taken place, the incidence rates approaching or surpassing those in whites in the same population and being three or four times higher than among Japanese in Japan.

Risk factors of a non-dietary origin

There is sufficient evidence that cigarette smoking and alcohol consumption are human carcinogens and that both lifestyle habits increases the risk of colorectal cancer. Evidence from observational studies indicates that long-term use of non-steroidal anti-inflammatory drugs (NSAIDS), including aspirin, may reduce the risk of colorectal cancer. Nevertheless, recommendations to general populations on NSAID or aspirin use for cancer prevention are premature given that use of these medications is accompanied by many side effects and may increase the risk of other serious medical conditions, necessitating close medical supervision. Thus, their use as chemopreventive agents may only be practical in those at very high risk of developing colorectal cancer (for example familial adenomatous polyposis (FAP) patients). In women, use of hormone replacement therapy (HRT) has been associated with a reduced risk of colorectal cancer but also with concomitant increases in the risk of breast cancer, and possibly coronary heart disease and thromboembolic events, making its use in any colorectal cancer prevention strategy impractical. Removal of adenomatous polyps has also been found to reduce disease risk, but in practice it is only applicable to those undergoing invasive screening.

Diet, dietary practices, nutrition and physical activity and colorectal cancer

The evidence of association between diet, dietary practices, nutrition and physical activity and colorectal cancer risk is, surprisingly, at times confusing and unclear.

ABC of Colorectal Cancer, Second Edition.
Edited by Annie Young, Richard Hobbs and David Kerr.
© 2011 Blackwell Publishing Ltd. Published 2011 by Blackwell Publishing Ltd.

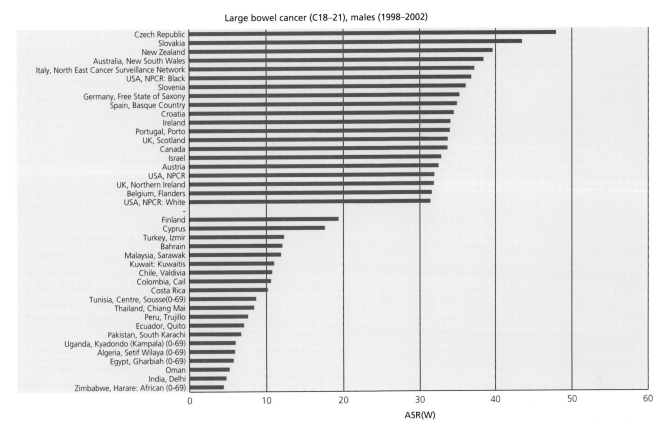

Figure 2.1 Highest and lowest incidence Age Standardised Rates (adjusted using the World Standard Population) (ASR(W)) for colorectal cancer worldwide for males.

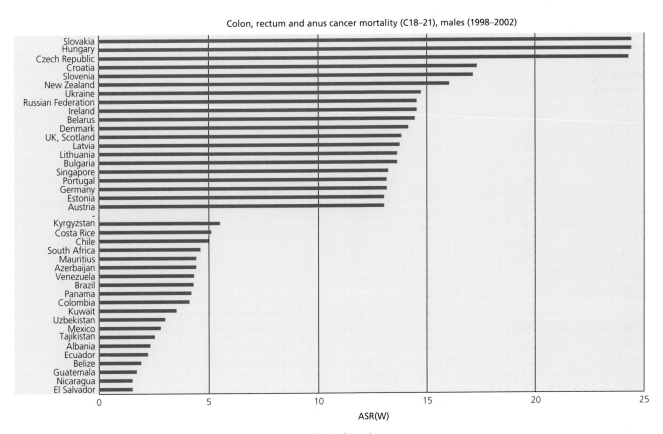

Figure 2.2 Highest and lowest mortality ASR(W) for colorectal cancer worldwide for males.

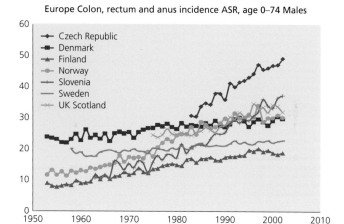

Figure 2.3 Trends on colorectal cancer incidence in Europe for selected countries (Nordcan; Socrates).

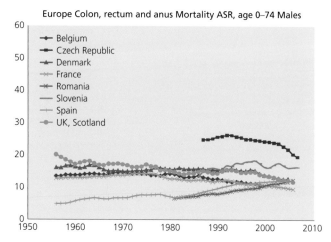

Figure 2.4 Trends on colorectal cancer mortality in Europe for selected countries (WHO mortality).

Physical activity

Evidence from epidemiological studies appears consistent that men with high occupational or recreational physical activity appear to be at a lower risk of colon cancer. Such evidence comes from follow-up studies of cohorts who are physically active or who have physically demanding jobs as well as case-control studies which have assessed physical activity by, for example, measurement of resting heart rate, or by questionnaire. Physical activity at a level equivalent to walking four hours per week has been associated with a decreased risk of colon cancer among women when compared to the sedentary group (RR = 0.62, 95% CI = 0.40–0.97).

Dietary pattern analysis

Dietary pattern analysis, based on the concept that foods eaten together are as important as a more reductive methodology characterised by a single food or nutrient analysis, has emerged as an alternative approach to study the relation between nutrition and diseases and tends to indicate that high consumption of fruits and vegetables and a low consumption of meat and saturated fatty

acids are associated with reduced colorectal cancer risk. However, there is some controversy surrounding these findings. For example, a meta-analysis of 13 prospective studies involving 3,635 cases of colorectal cancer and 459,910 participants found no association between total fat, saturated fat, monounsaturated fat and polyunsaturated fat consumption and colorectal cancer.

More than a decennia ago, fruits and vegetables were strongly and widely considered to reduce risk of colorectal cancer, a message strongly supported by the media. Many anticarcinogenic micronutrients, such as vitamin C, beta-carotene, folate, dietary fibre, flavonoids, selenium, phytosterols and other phytochemicals, have been proposed to contribute to this potential anticarcinogenic effect of fruits and vegetables.

In 1997, a World Cancer Research Fund/American Institute for Cancer Research report concluded that there was convincing evidence for a decreasing risk of colorectal cancer associated with increasing fruits and vegetable consumption. A decade later, in an updated report, the same organisation downgraded the protective effect of fruits and vegetables from *convincing* to *probable*. Between these reports, at the same time and using the same scientific evidence, an IARC Working Group declared a lack of association between consumption of fruits and vegetables and colorectal cancer.

Early cohort studies supported a protective effect for fruits and vegetables, which was not the case for more recent prospective research. Variations in results between cohort studies could be due to measurement error and to differences in adjustments. Most prospective studies used a single food frequency questionnaire to assess dietary exposition, which may not satisfactorily represent long-term intake.

In conclusion, the observed risk estimates in prospective studies between fruits, vegetables and colorectal cancer are very modest after adjustment for covariates.

Dietary fibre intake and colorectal cancer risk

Dietary fibre as an entity is difficult to separate from its dietary sources. Recent meta-analyses and pooled analyses have yielded null findings, that is no association between dietary fibre intake and colorectal cancer risk.

Red meat, processed meat and colorectal cancer

Prospective cohort and case-control studies have associated a daily intake of red and processed meat with an increased risk of colorectal cancer. The term red meat refers to beef, pork, lamb and goat; processed meat refers to meat preserved by smoking, curing, salting and/or addition of chemical preservatives. The results of meta-analysis support the hypothesis that high consumption of red and processed meat may increase the risk of colorectal cancer. However, the epidemiological association across the prospective studies is relatively weak with a 30% increased risk of colorectal cancer in high meat eaters compared to the lowest group of meat eaters.

Another hypothesis involves the potential role of nitrate and nitrite, commonly used in processed meats as preservation agents, as causes of human cancer. However, exposure is not specific to processed meat intake, as greater exposure may occur through consumption of other dietary sources such as vegetables or cereal products.

The formation of heterocyclic amines and polycyclic aromatic hydrocarbons in cooked meat has also been cited as a possible mechanism in the development of colorectal cancer. Heterocyclic amines and polycyclic aromatic hydrocarbons are carcinogenic in animal studies although evidence in humans is weak and inconsistent.

Finally, it has been suggested that iron, particularly haem iron, may play a role in colorectal cancer development. Red meat is a primary source of haem iron, which is found naturally in meat as part of haemoglobin and myoglobin, although relatively few studies have evaluated the potential role that this factor may play in cancer risk.

Vitamins and colorectal cancer

The use of multivitamin, vitamin D and folate supplements has been strongly correlated with healthy lifestyles, which could be associated with a lower risk of colorectal cancer. However, there is no compelling evidence to suggest that dietary supplementation is sufficiently worthwhile to be recommended.

Summary: lifestyle factors, dietary intakes and their consequences and colorectal cancer risk

Currently the weight of the existing evidence suggests that higher rates of smoking, alcohol consumption, intake of red/processed meats and reduced physical activity are all associated with increased risk of colorectal cancer.

Higher intake of fruits and vegetables may only moderately reduce the risk. A colorectal cancer preventive role of dietary or cereal fibre is debatable, despite recent findings suggesting a negative association with high intakes. Higher intake of calcium and vitamin D has been reported to be colorectal cancer protective, but except for modest findings for calcium supplementation in some intervention studies of adenoma recurrence, evidence is still lacking for any firm conclusions to be drawn. Much further research is required to elucidate the role of other compounds, foods, food components or their derivatives that may have effects that are colorectal cancer protective (folate, antioxidants, vitamins C and E, magnesium, selenium, phytochemicals, phytoestrogens, butyrate, resistant starches, tea/coffee, fish, whole grains, low glycemic index foods) or promotive (insulin, dietary carcinogens, secondary bile acids, iron, heterocyclic amines, refined sugars, high glycemic index foods). In addition, there are many complex interactions between environmental, dietary and genetic factors that may well modify colorectal cancer risk.

Among lifestyle factors, obesity has been suggested to be associated with an increased risk of colorectal cancer, although effects may vary by anatomical sub-site of the intestine and by gender. Physical inactivity has also been associated with an increased risk, although primarily for colon and less clearly for rectal cancer.

Thus, regular physical activity and avoidance of calorie over-consumption may represent two of the most effective ways of preventing this disease. Cigarette smoking is another major modifiable lifestyle factor that recent studies suggest is involved in the colorectal carcinogenesis process, although an induction period of four decades has been suggested.

As with many cancers, early detection of precancerous lesions and rapid, effective treatment of early colorectal tumours appear to be key points of screening and treatment strategies, not only for those at high risk of the disease, but also for general populations at large.

Nonetheless, the primarily sporadic nature of the disease indicates that a reduction in colorectal cancer incidence worldwide can best be achieved by effective primary prevention and changes in modifiable risk factors. Reducing cigarette consumption, decreasing alcohol intake, increasing physical activity and reducing consumption of red and processed meats could reduce the risk of colorectal cancer by more than one quarter.

Further reading

Alexander DD, Weed DL, Cushing CA, Lowe KA. Meta-analysis of prospective studies of red meat consumption and colorectal cancer. *Eur J Cancer Prev* (in press).

Autier P, Gandini S. Vitamin D supplementation and total mortality: a meta-analysis of randomized controlled trials. *Arch Intern Med* 2007 Sep;**167**(16):1730–1737.

Boyle P, Levin B (Eds) *World Cancer Report 2008*. IARC Press, Lyon (2009).

Boyle P, Boffetta P, Autier P. Diet, nutrition and cancer: public, media and scientific confusion. *Annals Oncol* 2008:191665–191667.

Ferlay J, Shin HR, Forman C, Mathers C, Parkin DM. GLOBOCAN 2008. *Cancer Incidence and Mortality Worldwide IARC Cancer Base*, 1027–5614; No. 10. Lyon, (2010).

CHAPTER 3

Pathways of Carcinogenesis

Michael Christie[1] and Oliver Sieber[2]

[1] Royal Melbourne Hospital, Melbourne, Australia
[2] Ludwig Institute for Cancer Research, Parkville, Australia

---

OVERVIEW

- Sporadic colorectal carcinogenesis is a multi-step evolutionary process
- Steps reflect advantageous mutations and epigenetic changes in tumour suppressor genes and oncogenes
- The changes that occur and the order in which they occur constitute the genetic pathways of carcinogenesis
- The majority of colorectal cancers develop along the classical histological adenoma-carcinoma sequence, which is associated with mutation of the *APC, KRAS, SMAD4* and *TP53* genes and often the acquisition of chromosomal instability
- A subset of colorectal carcinomas arise via a different genetic pathway characterised by mutation in the *BRAF* gene, CpG island hypermethylation at specific sites and the loss of DNA mismatch repair function resulting in hypermutation at repeat sequences including microsatellites (microsatellite instability); such cancers may arise via the serrated neoplasia sequence
- Genetic and epigenetic changes, individually and in combination, may determine disease prognosis and therapy response

---

Introduction

Carcinogenesis is the progressive, stepwise transformation of a normal cell into a malignant cancer cell (see Box 3.1, 'Hallmarks of cancer'). The 'steps' in this multi-step process are represented by genetic mutations or epigenetic changes that activate oncogenes or inactivate tumour suppressor genes and mutator genes (Table 3.1).

In their normal state, tumour suppressor genes inhibit cancer formation, but this inhibition is lost when both alleles (copies) of the gene are inactivated by (epi-) mutations. Given that 'two hits' are required to disrupt gene function, tumour suppressor genes are considered to act in a recessive fashion. Similarly, mutator genes normally maintain genomic integrity, but mutation results in a genome-wide increase in mutation rate (hypermutation), either in the form of specific types of small-scale mutations or large-scale chromosomal changes. In contrast, oncogenes promote

Box 3.1 **The hallmarks of cancer (Hanahan and Weinberg)**

- Self sufficiency in growth signals
- Insensitivity to growth-inhibitory signals
- Avoidance of apoptosis
- Limitless replicative potential
- Angiogenesis
- Invasion and metastasis

cancer formation when activated by mutations in one allele of the gene leading to excessive or inappropriate expression or excessive catalytic activity of the protein. Accordingly, oncogenes are said to act in a dominant fashion. The major tumour suppressor genes, oncogenes and mutator genes involved in colorectal cancer are summarised in Table 3.2.

The multi-step process of carcinogenesis is initiated by the occurrence of one or more mutations or epigenetic changes that give a cell a selective growth advantage (Figure 3.1). Analogous to Darwinian evolution, the clone derived from that cell then expands. Further progression to malignancy requires additional advantageous alterations, each of which is followed by a wave of clonal expansion. It is generally accepted that fully malignant behaviour only

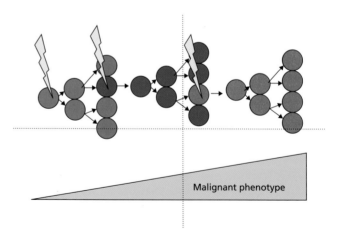

Figure 3.1 The somatic evolution of cancer. Tumour cells develop an increasingly malignant phenotype as they acquire successive selectively advantageous genetic mutation or epigenetic changes. (Epi-) mutations are followed by waves of clonal expansion.

ABC of Colorectal Cancer, Second Edition.
Edited by Annie Young, Richard Hobbs and David Kerr.
© 2011 Blackwell Publishing Ltd. Published 2011 by Blackwell Publishing Ltd.

Table 3.1 Types of genetic mutations and epigenetic changes in cancer.

Type of change	Effect on DNA	Effect on protein
Genetic: Small-scale mutation		
Point mutation	Exchange of a single nucleotide for another	Silent: coding for the same amino-acid Missense: coding for another amino acid Nonsense: creating a stop codon Splice site: removing or creating a splice site
Insertion/deletion	Addition/removal of one or more nucleotides	Frameshift: changing the reading frame of the protein In frame: adding/removing one or more amino acids Splice site: removing or creating a splice site
Genetic: Large-scale mutation		
Duplication/amplification	Gain of one or more copies of a large chromosomal region or a whole chromosome	Increase of dosage for single or multiple genes
Deletion	Loss of a large chromosomal region or a whole chromosome	Decrease of dosage for single or multiple genes Creation of novel fusion genes Aberrant gene expression in novel context
Translocation	Interchange between nonhomologous chromosomes	Creation of novel fusion genes Aberrant gene expression in novel context
Inversion	Reversing the orientation of a chromosomal segment	Creation of novel fusion genes Aberrant gene expression in novel context
Loss of heterozygosity	Loss of one allele, either by a deletion or recombination event	Reduction of two alleles to one allele for single or multiple genes
Epigenetic		
Addition or removal of methyl groups to DNA	At CpG sites, conversion of cytosine to 5-methylcytosine	Silencing or activation of gene expression
Modification of histone proteins	Acetylation, methylation, ubiquitylation, phosphorylation, sumoylation	Silencing or activation of gene expression

Table 3.2 Oncogenes and tumour suppressor genes commonly involved in sporadic colorectal cancer.

Gene name	Type of cancer gene	Frequency of mutation or epigenetic silencing	Consequences
APC	Tumour suppressor	~70%	Constitutive activation of the WNT signalling pathway
BRAF, KRAS	Oncogene	~10%, ~35%	Constitutive activation of the MAPK pathway
SMAD2, SMAD4, TGFBR2	Tumour suppressor	~5%, ~10%, ~15%	Decreased TGF-beta pathway signalling
TP53	Tumour suppressor	~50%	Impaired cellular stress and DNA damage response
MLH1	Mutator gene	~10%	Defective DNA mismatch repair

MAPK, mitogen activated protein kinase; TGF-beta, transforming growth factor-beta.

manifests once cells have acquired the capacity of self-sufficiency in growth signals, insensitivity to growth-inhibitory signals, avoidance of apoptosis, limitless replicative potential, angiogenesis, invasion and metastasis. The mutations and epigenetic changes which occur and the order in which they occur constitute the genetic pathways of carcinogenesis. The clonal evolution of colorectal cancer is reflected histologically by a sequence of premalignant lesions showing a progressive increase in atypia and eventually overt malignancy. Current evidence suggests that colorectal tumours develop along a limited number of alternative genetic pathways. The following discussion focuses on sporadic (non-familial) colorectal cancer. Familial colorectal cancer is discussed in Chapter 4.

The histological development of colorectal adenocarcinoma

The classical adenoma-carcinoma sequence

The development of most sporadic colorectal cancers from normal epithelium probably follows a relatively consistent histological sequence, the classical adenoma-carcinoma sequence (Figure 3.2). The first stage of this sequence is usually taken to be the onset of dysplasia involving a single crypt (unicryptal adenoma). Single dysplastic crypts develop into clusters of dysplastic crypts which grow to form adenomas that often change from a tubular to a tubulovillous or villous architecture as they increase in size. Similarly, the cells of adenomas show first mild, then moderate, and then severe cytological atypia. Eventually the defining features of malignancy (adenocarcinoma) appear; local invasion and metastasis to distant sites.

For sporadic colorectal tumours the progression from adenoma to carcinoma has been estimated to take approximately 10 to

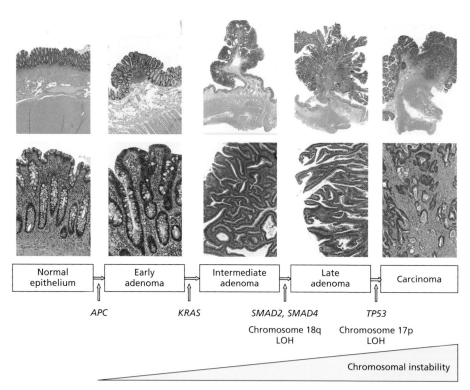

| Normal epithelium | → | Early adenoma | → | Intermediate adenoma | → | Late adenoma | → | Carcinoma |

APC   KRAS   SMAD2, SMAD4   TP53

Chromosome 18q LOH   Chromosome 17p LOH

Chromosomal instability

Figure 3.2 The classical adenoma-carcinoma sequence. Inactivation of the *APC* tumour suppressor gene results in defective Wnt signalling and initiates tumour formation. Subsequent progression towards malignancy is accompanied by mutation in the oncogene *KRAS*, loss of chromosome 18q harbouring the tumour suppressor genes *SMAD2* and *SMAD4*, and loss of chromosome 17p harbouring the tumour suppressor gene *TP53*. The extent of chromosomal instability increases with tumour progression. Villous morphology becomes more prominent as adenomas increase in size. The carcinoma is outlined in green.

40 years. However, there is evidence that not all adenomas undergo malignant transformation. For example, adenomas are considerably more frequent than carcinomas in the general population, taking into account that some patients will die before the adenomas have had sufficient time to progress to carcinoma. More direct evidence comes from long-term endoscopic studies demonstrating that some sporadic adenomas undergo spontaneous regression.

The serrated neoplasia sequence

In recent years, an alternative sequence of histopathological lesions leading to colorectal carcinoma has been identified, the serrated neoplasia sequence (Figure 3.3). Premalignant lesions in this sequence probably include two distinct types of serrated polyps, traditional serrated adenomas and sessile serrated adenomas, which together may constitute 5–10% of all polyps. However, the true magnitude of risk of progression to adenocarcinoma for these two types of polyps remains unknown and the recommendations on their clinical management continue to evolve. Compared to the classical adenoma-carcinoma sequence, the serrated neoplasia sequence appears to be associated with different sets of genetic and epigenetic changes. In particular, sessile serrated adenomas have been suggested to be possible precursor lesions for DNA mismatch repair deficient sporadic colorectal cancer (see below). The role of the pathologist in reporting such histology is outlined in Chapter 7.

Genetic pathways

The classical genetic pathway for sporadic colorectal cancer

Molecular studies of sporadic lesions from all stages of the classical adenoma-carcinoma sequence have uncovered a common

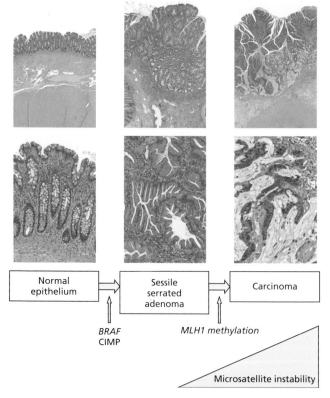

| Normal epithelium | → | Sessile serrated adenoma | → | Carcinoma |

BRAF CIMP   MLH1 methylation

Microsatellite instability

Figure 3.3 The serrated neoplasia sequence. Sessile serrated adenomas often show *BRAF* mutation and CpG island methylation at specific loci (CIMP). Progression to carcinoma may be associated with *MLH1* promoter hypermethylation and consequent impairment of DNA mismatch repair which manifests as microsatellite instability. Note the serrated luminal outlines in the sessile serrated adenoma, and the mucinous differentiation in the carcinoma.

succession of genetic and epigenetic changes in tumour suppressor genes and oncogenes (Figure 3.2). Tumour growth is probably most commonly initiated by bi-allelic mutation of the adenomatous polyposis coli (*APC*) tumour suppressor gene, with changes detectable in around 70% of microadenomas, early adenomas and carcinomas. *APC* is therefore often referred to as the gatekeeper of colorectal carcinogenesis. One consequence of *APC* mutation is aberrant activation of the Wnt signalling pathway, which plays a key role in controlling stem cell maintenance, proliferation and differentiation of colorectal epithelia.

Although bi-allelic *APC* mutation appears to trigger tumour formation, changes in additional genes are required for further adenoma growth and progression. Activating mutations in the v-Ki-ras2 Kirsten rat sarcoma viral oncogene homolog (*KRAS*), a member of the mitogen activated protein kinase (MAPK) pathway, are found at the transition from an early- to an intermediate-stage adenoma in around 35% of lesions.

Progression from an intermediate- to a late-stage adenoma is associated with loss of chromosome 18q, which is detected in around 60% of large adenomas. The two main tumour suppressor genes which are targeted by this loss are probably the SMAD family members 2 and 4 (*SMAD2* and *SMAD4*), both acting in the transforming growth factor-beta (TGF-beta) signalling pathway. Accordingly, mutations have been identified in *SMAD2* and *SMAD4* in sporadic colorectal cancers, albeit at a lower frequency than the chromosome 18q loss.

The transition from a late-stage adenoma to adenocarcinoma often coincides with loss of chromosome 17q, identifiable in around 50% of cases. The tumour protein p53 (*TP53*), a critical regulator of cellular stress and DNA damage responses, is the most likely target of this change. Chromosome 17q loss strongly correlates with missense and protein truncating mutations in *TP53*.

The cellular and genetic changes that lead to tumour invasion and metastasis are amongst the least understood aspects of colorectal cancer biology. Loss of E-cadherin function, a component of adherens-junctions between cells, is one of the aberrations which have been associated with cancer invasion.

Approximately 80% of colorectal cancers that develop along the classical pathway further appear to acquire some form of chromosomal instability, an increased rate of chromosomal gains, losses and/or rearrangements. However, around 20% of colorectal cancers maintain a relatively normal chromosomal karyotype with some data suggesting an overall better prognosis for patients with such tumours (see below).

DNA mismatch repair deficient sporadic colorectal cancer

Approximately 10–15% of sporadic colorectal cancers follow an alternative genetic pathway of carcinogenesis characterised by loss of DNA mismatch repair function. This defect is usually caused by hypermethylation of the mutL homolog 1 (MLH1) promoter resulting in silencing of transcription of this DNA mismatch repair gene. DNA mismatch repair deficiency results in genome-wide hypermutation at nucleotide repeat sequences including microsatellites, short tandem repeat sequences of 1–6 base-pairs of DNA.

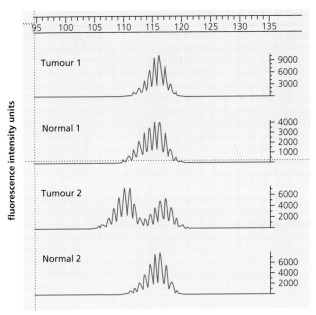

PCR fragment size in base pairs

Figure 3.4 Microsatellite instability in colorectal cancer as indicated by fragment analysis of the mononucleotide repeat marker BAT26. The microsatellite marker BAT26 has been PCR-amplified from tumour and normal DNA from two patients using fluorescently-labelled primers. The PCR-products have been separated according to size. Tumour 2 shows an additional BAT26 peak due to a 6 base-pair deletion within the mononucleotide repeat. In clinical practice, a panel of 5 microsatellite markers, the Bethesda panel (BAT25, BAT26, D5S346 and D17S250), is generally analysed. A tumour is classified as microsatellite unstable if two or more of the five loci show instability.

Microsatellite instability (MSI) detected by polymerase chain reaction (PCR) amplification is a commonly used marker for such tumours (Figure 3.4). In addition, these tumours tend to accumulate frameshift mutations within coding repeats of certain cancer genes including axin 2 (*AXIN2*), transforming growth factor beta receptor II (*TGFBR2*), insulin-like growth factor 2 receptor (*IGF2R*), BCL2-associated X protein (*BAX*) and E2F transcription factor 4 (*E2F4*). Selectively neutral bystander mutations in coding repeats of other genes are also common.

DNA mismatch repair deficient tumours further tend to display activating point mutations in the v-raf murine sarcoma viral oncogene homolog B1 (*BRAF*), and CpG island hypermethylation at specific loci, a phenomenon referred to as CpG island methylator phenotype (CIMP). The chromosomal karyotype of these tumours tends to be normal, suggesting that microsatellite instability and chromosomal instability are mutually exclusive.

Intriguingly, sporadic cancers with defective DNA mismatch repair show clinicopathological features distinct from other sporadic colorectal cancers. MSI-positive cancers are associated with female gender, older age, right sided location and several histopathological features including mucinous differentiation, higher grade (poor differentiation) and a pronounced lymphocytic infiltrate. The presence of MSI has been associated with better disease prognosis and lack of response to fluorouracil (5-FU) based chemotherapy (see below). Notably, sessile serrated adenomas appear to share many of the molecular and clinical characteristics

Table 3.3 Prognostic and predictive factors in colorectal cancer.

Marker	Predictive significance	Prognostic significance
KRAS mutation	Confirmed to predict a lack of response to anti-EGFR antibody therapy*	–
BRAF mutation	May predict a lesser response to anti-EGFR antibody therapy	May indicate a worse prognosis in patients with metastatic disease
Microsatellite instability (DNA mismatch repair deficiency)	May predict a lesser response to fluorouracil, and an improved response to irinotecan	May indicate a better prognosis
Aneuploidy/Polyploidy (Chromosomal instability)	–	May indicate a worse prognosis

*Only *KRAS* mutation status is currently recommended as a marker for clinical use. EGFR, epidermal growth factor receptor

of MSI-positive carcinomas, suggesting that these may be the corresponding precursor lesions in a proportion of cases.

(Epi-) Mutations, disease prognosis and therapy response

There is increasing evidence that certain mutations or epigenetic changes are associated with disease prognosis (prognostic markers) and/or response to therapy (predictive markers) (Table 3.3). Although the use of molecular genetic changes as prognostic or predictive markers for colorectal cancer is currently limited with very few clinical applications, this field is expected to expand in the coming years. See Chapter 4, Clinical Genetics in the Management of Colon Cancer.

The best example of a clinically useful predictive marker is *KRAS* mutation which predicts resistance to anti-epidermal growth factor receptor (EGFR) antibody therapy, mostly used to treat patients with metastatic colorectal cancer. Current recommendations are that all colorectal cancer patients being considered for such therapy should have *KRAS* mutation testing performed on tumour samples, and only patients lacking *KRAS* mutation should receive anti-EGFR antibody therapy. *BRAF* mutation may similarly predict a lack of response to anti-EGFR therapy, but this latter association remains a subject of investigation.

Genomic instability status is also a marker of potential prognostic and predictive value, although it is not yet used in the clinic. Studies indicate that MSI-positive cancers have a better prognosis than MSI-negative cancers, may not benefit from adjuvant 5-FU based therapy, but may show an improved response to irinotecan based therapy. Similarly chromosomal instability (aneuploidy/polyploidy) appears to be associated with a worse prognosis.

Current research aims to further characterise the associations of genetic and epigenetic changes, individually and in combination, with disease prognosis and therapy response. This work may ultimately lead to the development of molecular signatures which may in the future allow more rational planning of treatment and follow-up. As novel therapies targeting mutant proteins in cancer are being developed, mutation testing to select patients for treatment will become more commonplace.

Further reading

Boland CR, Goel A. Microsatellite instability in colorectal cancer. *Gastroenterology* 2010;**138**:2073–2087.e3.

Fearon ER, Vogelstein B. A genetic model for colorectal tumorigenesis. *Cell* 1990;**61**:759–767.

Hanahan D, Weinberg RA. The hallmarks of cancer. *Cell* 2000;**100**:57–70.

Jass JR. Classification of colorectal cancer based on correlation of clinical, morphological and molecular features. *Histopathology* 2007;**50**:113–130.

Markowitz SD, Bertagnolli MM. Molecular origins of cancer: Molecular basis of colorectal cancer. *N Engl J Med* 2009;**361**:2449–2460.

Walther A, Johnstone E, Swanton C, Midgley R, Tomlinson I, Kerr D. Genetic prognostic and predictive markers in colorectal cancer. *Nat Rev Cancer* 2009:1–11.

CHAPTER 4

Clinical Genetics in the Management of Colon Cancer

Kai Ren Ong[1], *Vicky Bowyer*[2] *and Trevor Cole*[1]

[1]Birmingham Women's NHS Foundation Trust, Birmingham, UK
[2]Health Sciences Research Institute, Warwick Medical School, The University of Warwick, Coventry, UK

OVERVIEW

- The majority of individuals with a family history of colorectal cancer will themselves be at near population risk of developing cancer

- Recognition of a possible familial colorectal cancer syndrome is the key to management

- Treatment includes genetic counselling, genetic testing and screening for cancer

- There is evidence that surveillance programmes are effective in reducing colorectal cancer mortality in dominantly inherited colorectal cancer syndromes

- A carefully designed standard protocol to collect family history information at primary care level facilitates appropriate rapid referral to screening units, genetics services or back to primary care

Introduction

Before 1990, the role of inherited factors in the aetiology of adult cancer was relatively poorly understood and aroused little interest among doctors and the public alike – although familial adenomatous polyposis (the autosomal dominant colon cancer syndrome referred to in the previous chapter) was an exception in this respect. However, in the last 20 years interest has increased markedly. In the West Midlands (population 5.5 million), for example, familial cancer referrals constituted 1% of all clinical genetic referrals in 1991, whereas now they represent 41% of cases (3,635 cases in 2009) (Figure 4.1).

Despite the estimate that 5–10% of colorectal cancer has an inherited basis, only a small percentage of referred families have mutations in one of the currently identified genes. Furthermore, mutation studies are usually possible only if DNA is available from an affected patient, so molecular investigation will facilitate the management of only a small number of cases. The remaining referrals must be managed with clinically derived strategies. This article discusses the clinical features and management of dominant colon cancer syndromes and provides referral guidelines and screening protocols for more common familial clusters.

Genetic counselling for families with a history of cancer requires a full and accurate family history. When possible, histological confirmation of the reported tumours should be obtained. It should then be possible to recognise the specific cancer syndromes. It is important to emphasise to families that however extensive the family history of cancer, (unless present on both sides), the patient will always have a greater than 50% chance of *not* developing that particular tumour. This simple fact is often overlooked and may surprise but greatly reassure many patients.

Familial adenomatous polyposis (FAP)

FAP, previously called polyposis coli (or Gardners syndrome if extra colonic manifestations were present, Figure 4.2 and 4.3), is the best recognised of the colorectal cancer syndromes but accounts for less than 1% of all colorectal cancers and has a prevalence of 1 in 14,000. It is characterised by the presence of 100 or more tubo-villous adenomas in the colon, with intervening micro-adenoma on histological examination. The mean age of diagnosis of polyps is during teenage years, and almost all of gene carriers have polyps by the age of 40. If these are left untreated, malignant transformation is inevitable with a mean age of colorectal cancer occurring during the patient's mid-30s, often with synchronous tumours.

This condition is an autosomal dominant disorder, therefore the offspring of affected individuals are at a 50% risk of being gene carriers. The diagnosis of FAP should always result in a careful and full evaluation of the family history. Wherever possible, parents should have at least one colonoscopy, irrespective of age. In most cases without a family history, parental examination will be negative and the proband (the subject being studied or reported on) will probably be one of 30% of cases that represent new mutations. However the siblings of all probands should be offered annual colonoscopy up to the age of 30, reducing to 3 yearly intervals until aged 60 or until proven to be non-gene carriers.

The cloning of the causative gene (APC) on chromosome 5 in 1991 dramatically changed the management of FAP. If DNA is available from an affected individual, sequencing will detect mutations in 99% of families with classical FAP. In these families first-degree relatives should be offered predictive testing with appropriate genetic

ABC of Colorectal Cancer, Second Edition.
Edited by Annie Young, Richard Hobbs and David Kerr.
© 2011 Blackwell Publishing Ltd. Published 2011 by Blackwell Publishing Ltd.

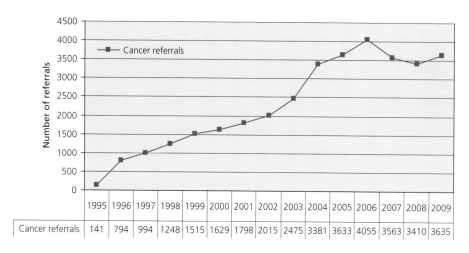

| Cancer referrals | 141 | 794 | 994 | 1248 | 1515 | 1629 | 1798 | 2015 | 2475 | 3381 | 3633 | 4055 | 3563 | 3410 | 3635 |

Figure 4.1 Number of referrals of patients with cancer to West Midlands Regional Clinical Genetics Service, 1995–2009.

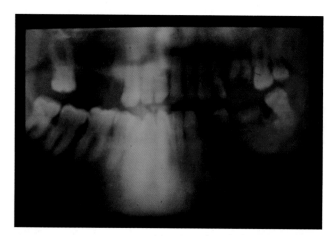

Figure 4.2 Mandibular cysts in Familial Adenomatous Polyposis.

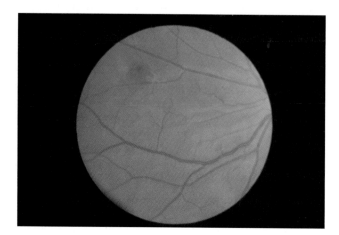

Figure 4.3 Congenital hypertrophy of the retinal pigment epithelium (CHRPE) in Familial Adenomatous Polyposis.

counselling. In families with no identified mutation, linkage studies to identify the 'high risk' chromosome 5 are possible in many cases. Non-gene carriers should be reassured and surveillance stopped. Gene carriers should be offered annual surveillance from the age of 12. Once a number of polyps are identified, the timing and type of

surgery available should be discussed (a sensitive issue in teenagers and young adults). The two most common options are ileal-rectal anastomosis and annual surveillance of the remaining rectal tissue or alternatively an ileal-anal anastomosis and reconstruction of a rectal pouch using terminal small bowel.

Molecular testing is usually offered to 'at risk' children at ages of 10–14 before starting annual sigmoidoscopy. However, parental pressure for earlier testing (prior to the child being able to give consent), is not uncommon and the timing of testing continues to be a subject of debate.

Cloning APC explained several clinical features and aided studies of genotypes and phenotypes. For example the presence of congenital hypertrophy of the retinal pigment epithelium (Figure 4.3), an attenuated phenotype, (that is, fewer than 100 polyps or late onset) and non-malignant but debilitating and potentially lethal desmoid disease each show an association with mutations in specific exon regions. The cloning also confirmed clinical findings that FAP and Gardner's syndrome were different manifestations of the same disease spectrum that could coexist within the same family.

With greater clinical awareness, regular surveillance and the advent of molecular investigation, almost all colorectal cancer deaths in inherited cases of FAP can be avoided. Increased survival has revealed later complications, in particular periampullary or duodenal adenocarcinoma (occurring in 2–12% of individuals post-colectomy). Also important are aggressive desmoid disease and other rarer malignant diseases (Box 4.1).

Box 4.1 **Early and late extracolonic tumours in familial adenomatous polyposis**

Hepatoblastoma (early)
Adrenal adenoma (early or late)
Desmoid disease (early or late)
Papillary thyroid cancer – predominantly females (late)
Periampullary carcinoma (late)

Multi-centre studies of chemoprophylactic approaches to reduce polyp growth (for example, aspirin and non-digestible starch) are in the follow-up phase at present.

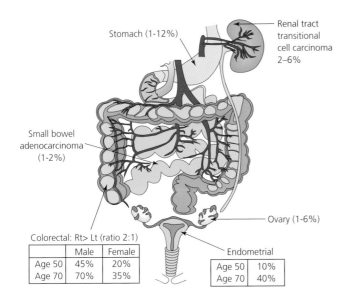

Figure 4.4 Tumours in hereditary non-polyposis colorectal cancer (upper figure in ranges may be overestimates due to ascertainment bias).

Colorectal: Rt> Lt (ratio 2:1)

	Male	Female
Age 50	45%	20%
Age 70	70%	35%

Age 50	10%
Age 70	40%

Lynch syndrome

Lynch syndrome (LS), also known as hereditary non-polyposis colon cancer (HNPCC), became more widely recognised about 30 years ago in families manifesting mainly colorectal cancer segregating in an autosomal dominant fashion. Many families also exhibit extra-colonic tumours, particularly gynaecological, small bowel or urinary tract carcinomas (Figure 4.4) and these became known as Lynch type 2 to distinguish them from site specific colorectal cancer families, designated Lynch type 1. The subsequent name change to HNPCC was potentially misleading as many gene carriers will develop a small number of tubo-villous adenomas, but not more than 100 as seen in FAP, and Lynch syndrome has become the preferred name again. The proportion of CRC due to LS is controversial and estimates range from 1% to 20%; most observers, however, suggest about 2%.

The diagnosis of LS is suspected on the basis of the family history, as the appearance of the bowel, unlike FAP, is a not diagnostic. To improve the recognition of LS, diagnostic criteria were devised in Amsterdam in 1991 and were subsequently amended to include non-colonic tumours (Box 4.2). Confirmation of the diagnosis is usually through molecular testing.

Mutations in four mismatch repair (MMR) genes, *MLH1*, *MSH2*, *MSH6* and *PMS2* have been linked with LS. If both copies of the genes are mutated, as postulated in Knudson's two hit hypothesis, that cell and all its daughter cells are missing a vital mechanism for repair of DNA in somatic tissue. Molecular studies showed that a

significant minority (approximately 30%) of early onset CRC (less than 35 years) is due to mutations in the MMR genes. Mutations in the MMR genes lead to microsatellite instability (MSI) (Figure 4.5) and loss of expression of the MMR proteins in the tumour tissue (Figure 4.6). MSI is the presence of additional alleles of certain short tandem-repeat DNA sequences ('microsatellites') – see Chapter 3 Pathways of Carcinogenesis, and is present in more than 90% of LS related colorectal tumours. Loss of MMR protein expression may be detected using immunohistochemistry (IHC). The finding of MSI and MMR protein loss is a strong indicator that a mutation in a MMR gene is present, and MSI and IHC studies on stored tumour tissue are now routinely used to select cases for germline mutation testing.

Risk estimates vary widely across different studies, with lifetime risks of, for example, male bowel cancer ranging from below 50% to almost 100% (Table 4.1). This reflects differences in ascertainment of the families, age at the end of follow-up and methods of statistical analysis. However, consensus approximate lifetime risks of developing the main LS related cancers are shown in Figure 4.4, and these are frequently quoted during the counselling of families.

A review by Lindor *et al.* in 2006 found evidence suggesting that screening for colorectal cancer in LS is beneficial in reducing mortality. Previously, Vasen *et al.* (1999) had reported that screening is cost-effective. The method of choice is colonoscopy rather than flexible sigmoidoscopy as 80% of cancers are proximal to the rectum compared to only 57% in sporadic CRC. Failure to reach the caecum should be followed by barium enema examination, although surveillance using radiological techniques should probably be used sparingly due to the theoretical mutagenic consequences in patients with DNA repair defects. However, the optimal surveillance frequency is controversial. Recent guidelines recommend 2 yearly screening, but interval cancers have been reported, suggesting that screening should perhaps be more frequent than this. Patients should understand that the strategy of colonoscopy is the removal of polyps and prevention of tumours or early diagnosis, but that complete prevention is impossible. Extra-colonic screening guidelines are summarised in Box 4.3 and Table 4.2.

Table 4.1 Penetrance of colorectal and endometrial cancers in LS in different studies.

	Colorectal cancer penetrance (%)		Length of follow-up	Endometrial cancer penetrance (%)	Length of follow-up
	Males	Females			
Hampel *et al.* 2005	68.7	52.2	Lifetime	54	Lifetime
Aarnio *et al.* 1999	100	54	To 70yr	60	To 70yr
Quehenberger *et al.* 2005	26.7	22.4	To 70yr	31.5	To 70yr

Tumour

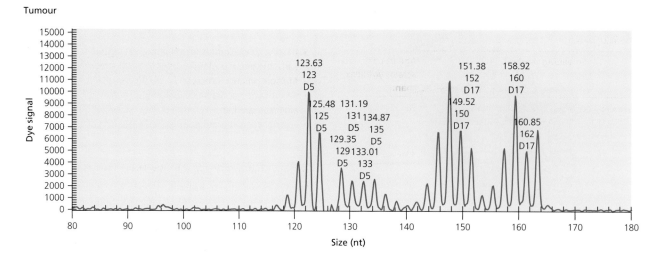

Normal

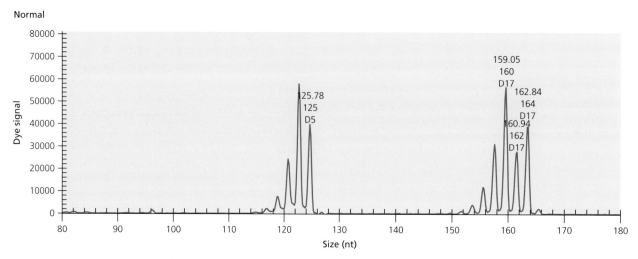

Figure 4.5 Microsatellite instability. The upper figure shows extra peaks representing additional alleles of the microsatellite marker present in the tumour, which are absent in the patient's normal tissue (lower figure).

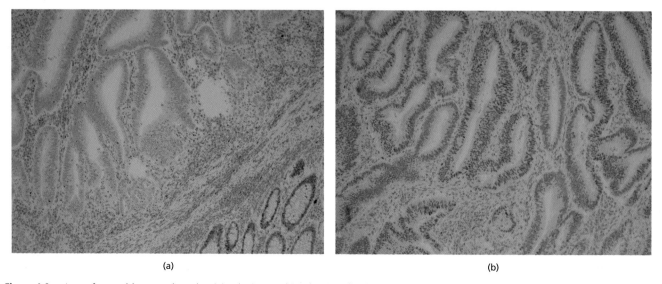

Figure 4.6 a. Loss of normal brown coloured staining by immunohistochemistry for the MSH2 protein in colon carcinoma cells which are blue in colour. b. Normal preservation of protein staining in colon cancer.

Table 4.2 Guidelines of the international workshop on surveillance in Lynch Syndrome, convened in 2006 (summarised in Vasen et al., JMG 2007, 44; 353–362). Evidence of benefit is still not available.

Site	Screening method	Age at first screen not later than:
Endometrium	Gynaecological exam, transvaginal ultrasound and aspiration biopsy 1–2 yrly	30–35yr
Ovary	Transvaginal ultrasound 1–2-yrly Measurement of serum Ca 125	30–35yr
Stomach	Gastroscopy 1–2 yrly in those with a family history of gastric cancer	30–35yr
Urinary tract	Renal ultrasound, cystoscopy, urine analysis and cytology 1–2 yrly in those with a family history of renal or urinary tract cancers	30–35yr

Box 4.3 **Screening of other organs in LS**

- Screening of other organ systems has not yet been proven to be beneficial
- However, screening for gynaecological tumours in mutation positive families is widely offered, irrespective of the family history, as 40% of female gene carriers develop endometrial carcinomas
- If tumours have previously been identified within the family in the gynaecological or urinary tract, surveillance also offered

Familial clusters with no recognisable single gene disorder

Families whose cancers do not meet the diagnostic criteria of FAP, LS or rarer colorectal cancer syndromes (such as syndromes related to the PTEN gene, MYH gene, Turcot syndrome, Peutz-Jegher syndrome or Juvenile polyposis) make up the largest and most difficult group of patients requesting management. There is rarely any indication of the aetiological basis of the cluster of colorectal cancer and many instances will be coincidental occurrences. Other tumour clusters may be due to common environmental exposures, the effect of multiple low penetrance genes or an interaction of both these elements. The risk of colorectal cancer may be assessed using empiric risk figures (Table 4.3). These figures are estimates, however, and do not take into account factors such as the number of unaffected relatives. Further enquiry is usually justified if features

Table 4.3 Lifetime risk of colorectal cancer in first degree relatives of patient with colorectal cancer (from Houlston et al., 1990).

Population risk	1 in 50
One first degree relative affected (any age)	1 in 17
One first degree and one second degree relative affected	1 in 12
One first degree relative affected (age <45)	1 in 10
Two first degree relatives affected	1 in 6
Autosomal dominant pedigree	1 in 2

Box 4.4 **Four pointers to recognition of familial cancer clusters**

- High frequency of the same tumour in the family
- Early age of onset of tumours
- Multiple primary tumours
- Recognised associations – for example, colorectal and endometrial adenocarcinomas

such as multiple relatives with the same tumour or early onset of tumours are present in a family (Box 4.4).

Concerns that it is often impossible to provide precise risk figures may be misguided, as there is evidence that many patients have difficulty interpreting risk figures and often are only requesting general guidance on risk and a discussion of management options. However, many different screening protocols have been suggested in the past and the lack of consistency and long-term audit in these families is a problem.

To manage familial cancer in the West Midlands, a protocol has been developed which maximises the role of primary care (Figure 4.7). The protocol provides clear inclusion and screening guidelines for cancer units and centres. This has promoted a consistency of management across families as well as between families and is now allowing collection of data for audit. Table 4.4 summarises the recent recommendations for screening commissioned by the British Society of Gastroenterology and the Association of Coloproctology for Great Britain and Ireland. These are useful guidelines but advice from a tertiary genetics unit should be sought for apparently moderate and high risk families, as additional molecular investigations may help to tailor surveillance more appropriately. In particular, some families may benefit from individual clinical or molecular evaluation and modification of the advice given in the guidelines.

The issue of whether primary care should use a reactive or proactive approach is still debated. In the West Midlands, patients requesting advice are asked to complete a family history questionnaire at home. This form and the inclusion criteria are available at http://www.bwhct.nhs.uk/genetics-wmfacs-documents.htm. Completion of the form in the patient's own time, at home, facilitates discussion with relatives to clarify the relevant information and saves time if a referral is required.

After histological confirmation in suspected familial cases, the data are evaluated centrally to identify high risk families requiring specialist investigation or referral to a screening unit. In a pilot study (population 200,000) the protocol reduced referrals from primary care by 50% with a greater reduction in screening due to a fall in low risk referrals to cancer units. This was associated with an increased referral rate for high risk referrals to clinical genetics. Central coordination prevents unnecessary reinvestigations for different branches of any one family.

Reports from local screening units and primary care suggest that the system of triage is beneficial in optimising screening efficiency. Further studies of patient satisfaction and how best to provide reassurance would be valuable.

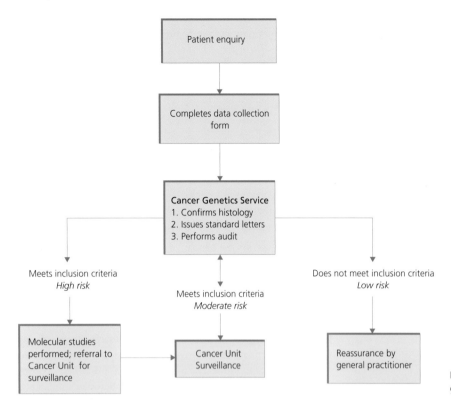

Figure 4.7 West Midlands protocol for cancer genetics referrals.

Table 4.4 The guidelines for colorectal screening summarised from Cairns *et al. Gut* 2010. Microsatellite instability studies and immunohistochemistry for loss of mismatch repair proteins may aid in the modification of these guidelines for individual families. All individuals should be encouraged to participate in population screening programmes as they are made available.

Family history	Screening regime
FAP – 50% risk no mutation	Colorectal – annual surveillance starting 13–15yrs until 30, then 3–5 yrly from 30–60 Upper GI – 3 yrly OGD from 30
FAP – known mutation	Annual surveillance until surgery
Lynch Syndrome: family members at 50% risk (where no mutation has been found but family meets Amsterdam criteria) and proven gene carriers	Colonoscopy 2 yearly (discuss 18 monthly) from 25–70/75 Upper GI – if family history of gastric cancer, 2 yrly OGD from 50 until 75
Colon cancer family histories*	
3 any age but all >50yrs 2 < 60 or mean <60yrs	'High Moderate' – 5 yrly 50–75
1 < 50yrs 2 between 60–70yrs 2 > 70yrs	'Low Moderate' – one colonoscopy at 55

OGD – oesophago-gastro-duodenoscopy
*Relatives should be first degree relatives of each other and of the proband

Acknowedgements

We would like to thank Kerry Wall and Jennie Bell from the West Midlands Regional Genetics Laboratory and Philippe Taniere, Consultant Histopathologist, University Hospital Birmingham NHS Trust for their assistance.

Further reading

Cairns SR *et al.* Guidelines for colorectal cancer screening and surveillance in moderate and high risk groups (update from 2002). *Gut* 2010;**59**: 666–689.

Foulkes W. A tale of four syndromes: familial adenomatous polyposis, Gardner syndrome, attenuated APC and Turcots syndrome. *QJM* 1995;**88**:853–863.

Hodgson, SV, Foulkes, WD, Eng, C, Maher, ER (Eds) *A Practical Guide to Human Cancer Genetics*. Cambridge University Press, 2007.

Houlston RS, Murday V, Harcocopos C, Williams CB, Slack J. Screening and genetic counselling for relatives of patients with colorectal cancer in a family cancer clinic. *BMJ* 1990;**301**:18–25.

Vasen HFA *et al.* Guidelines for the clinical management of Lynch syndrome (hereditary non-polyposis cancer) *J Med Genet* 2007;**44**:353–362.

CHAPTER 5

Screening for Colorectal Cancer

Julietta Patnick[1] *and Wendy S. Atkin*[2]

[1]NHS Cancer Screening Programmes, Oxford University, UK
[2]Imperial College London, London, UK

OVERVIEW

- People living in the UK have a 1 in 20 chance of developing colorectal cancer

- Survival is only 50% if diagnosed in people with symptoms but over 90% if detected at an early localised stage

- Screening for early colorectal cancer can reduce colorectal cancer mortality. Finding and removing adenomas from which cancers slowly develop reduces incidence as well as mortality

- Randomised trials have shown that colorectal cancer mortality can be reduced by 2-yearly faecal occult blood testing (FOBt) and by once only flexible sigmoidoscopy

- Other methods for screening which have not been tested in randomised trials include faecal immunochemical testing, colonoscopy, CT colonography

- The English Bowel Cancer Screening Programme offers 2-yearly screening by FOBt to people aged 60–74 and will shortly be introducing flexible sigmoidoscopy screening for those in their mid to late 50s. FOBt screening is currently available in Wales and Northern Ireland to those aged 60–69 and in Scotland to those aged 50–74

Approximately 21,000 men and around 18,000 women are diagnosed with colorectal cancer each year in the United Kingdom. It is the third most common cancer after lung and breast cancer and the second most common cause of cancer death, killing over 16,000 people each year.

Survival rates have doubled over the past 30 years, and are now at 50% for both colon and rectal cancer, with rates slightly higher in women than in men. However, it has long been known that survival varies by stage at diagnosis. Someone diagnosed with the earliest stage, a Duke's A colorectal cancer, has a greater than 90% chance of surviving more than 5 years; this drops to around 5% if the cancer has spread to other parts of the body (Duke's D) – see Table 7.1 in Chapter 7. It is this survival differential that led to the initial interest in screening the large bowel. In addition,

since colorectal cancers are thought to develop over a long period from adenomatous polyps in the bowel wall, it was suggested that finding and removing such polyps through screening could lead to a reduction in the incidence of colorectal cancer.

Many countries throughout the world have introduced colorectal cancer screening following publication of the results of faecal occult blood test (FOBt) trials in the 1990s. Most screening programmes therefore use the FOBt and a few use endoscopic methods.

How does the current colorectal cancer screening programme work in the UK?

England was the first of the UK countries to introduce a screening programme for people at average risk of colorectal cancer. Following an extensive pilot in England and Scotland, which operated from 2000, the screening programme in England started in 2006.

In England the programme initially targeted those aged 60–69, but now that it is operational across the country, it is extending to reach all people aged 60–74 inclusive. It uses the guaiac FOBt and is modelled on the Nottingham trial protocol which was replicated in the UK pilot.

The programme operates five 'hubs' which send invitations and literature to the target population, followed shortly afterwards by a FOBt kit. This comprises three cards of two windows each on to which the subject is asked to place a faecal smear sample from each of three bowel motions (Figure 5.1). This card is then returned by post to the hub in a plastic lined envelope. At the hub it is developed and the results are sent to the subject and his/her GP. Currently acceptance rates are just over 50%.

If the test is positive, the patient is sent an appointment to visit a screening centre. If the test is 'weakly positive', the subject is asked to repeat the test once or twice until a decision to refer to a screening centre or return to routine screening is made. About 2% of subjects who complete a test are referred.

The screening centres are accredited local endoscopy centres. After a positive FOBt the patient is first counselled and their health status checked. If appropriate, colonoscopy is offered and the need for careful bowel preparation explained. Around 10% of patients who have a positive FOB test and undergo colonoscopy are found to have an invasive cancer present. Of the rest, half have adenomas found and of the remainder some will have other bowel pathology. Around one third will have a normal colon.

ABC of Colorectal Cancer, Second Edition.
Edited by Annie Young, Richard Hobbs and David Kerr.
© 2011 Blackwell Publishing Ltd. Published 2011 by Blackwell Publishing Ltd.

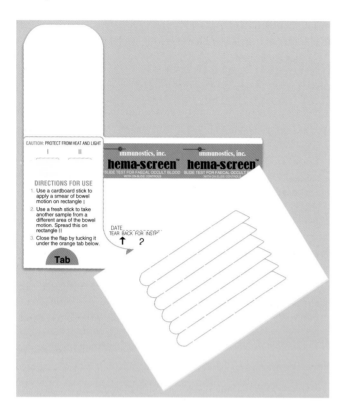

Figure 5.1 FOBt kit and application sticks.

In Northern Ireland and Wales the colorectal cancer screening programmes are currently only inviting those aged 60–69, although the Welsh Assembly government has announced the intention to extend its programme to age 74 by 2015. In Scotland, FOBT screening is available now to those aged 50–74. In each of these three countries there is a single 'hub' providing call and recall and laboratory services. One difference between the protocols in these countries and in England is that instead of asking the participant to repeat a weakly positive test, an immunochemical test is used as a reflex test on unprocessed faecal smears supplied on the same occasion by the participant. There are other slight differences in the methods of referral from hub to centre in the three countries and in the selection of endoscopists and endoscopy centres.

What is the evidence for FOBt?

Four randomised controlled trials of using a guaiac FOBt took place during the 1970s and 1980s. A Cochrane review published in 2007 put together the results of these trials and concluded that on an 'intention to treat' basis, two yearly screening with guaiac FOBt resulted in a 15% reduction in mortality from colorectal cancer in an invited population aged 50–69. When considered on a 'per protocol', or participation basis, this rose to 25%.

Only one of the trials, the Minnesota trial, showed any reduction in incidence. This trial rehydrated the guaiac in the laboratory in order to improve sensitivity. This in turn increased the positivity rate so that, after several rounds of screening, around 30% of trial participants needed to have a colonoscopy. After 18 years of follow up, incidence was reduced by 17% in those who underwent

2-yearly screening. In the other trials, which did not rehydrate the test, only 4% required a colonoscopy and no reduction in incidence occurred.

What other screening methods are used?

Immunochemical FOBt

The guaiac FOBt identifies intermittent bleeding from cancers and large adenomas in the bowel and is generally accepted to be only 50–60% sensitive. In addition, it can be positive when the subject has recently consumed rare meat, beetroot or other substances which contain haem. A more modern FOB test is the immunochemical test, sometimes called the iFOBt or the Faecal Immunochemical Test (FIT). This test is positive only for human globin present in the large bowel and is unaffected by diet. As it is a quantified test, the positivity level, and thus the sensitivity/specificity balance, can be controlled. This feeds directly onto the workload for colonoscopy. Immunochemical tests are commercially available and are used in screening programmes in a variety of countries. They have not been tested in a randomised trial setting.

Flexible sigmoidoscopy

Flexible sigmoidoscopy is an endoscopic procedure which examines the distal bowel (rectum and sigmoid colon) where around half of adenomas and cancers are located (Figure 5.2). Most people who are destined to develop cancer in the distal bowel will have developed a distal adenoma by the time they reach their mid to late 50s. With this in mind, a number of trials have been designed to look at the effectiveness of a single flexible sigmoidoscopy examination between the ages of 55 and 64. Some early results were published from the Norwegian trial, but the first definitive results were published in May 2010. These were from the UK trial and showed, after 11 years of follow-up, a reduction in colorectal cancer mortality of 32% on an 'intention to treat' basis (among those invited to do the test), and 43% on a 'per protocol' basis (among those who had the test done). There was also a reduction in incidence of 23% and 33% correspondingly. In the distal bowel incidence of cancer was reduced by 50% in those screened. Flexible sigmoidoscopy is

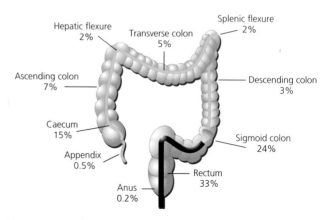

Figure 5.2 Site of cancers in the bowel and the usual reach of screening flexible sigmoidoscopy.

attractive for the patient since it requires only a self-administered enema not full bowel cleansing, sedation is not usually required and the recovery time is much less. Most people can have their polyps removed during the screening, although 1 in 20 have higher risk adenomas and are offered colonoscopy to screen the proximal colon.

Colonoscopy

Optical colonoscopy is often seen as the 'gold standard' screening test since it enables full examination of the entire colon and removal of any polyps or biopsy of any mass in one procedure (Figure 5.3). It takes more time for the endoscopist than flexible sigmoidoscopy and requires more support staff and facilities and greater commitment from the patient. The relative benefits and harms of colonoscopy as a screening technique have not been tested in a randomised trial; nevertheless in the USA, the United States Preventative Services Task Force (USPSTF) recommends colonoscopy once every 10 years for adults aged 50 or older as one of a range of screening modalities and it is also available as a screening test under national schemes in Poland and Germany.

CT Colonography

CT Colonography (CTC) is the preferred imaging modality for patients who are deemed unsuitable for optical colonoscopy, and there are patients who might prefer this as their first line investigation. It is gradually replacing barium enema as equipment and expertise becomes more available. It has been shown to be almost as sensitive as optical colonoscopy for larger polyps, with 90% sensitivity for ≥ 10 mm and 78% for ≥ 6 mm polyps. The perforation rate of CTC is much less than for OC, but a second procedure is necessary for those in whom some pathology is found, which increases the cost of screening using CTC. It has not yet been subject to a randomised trial for screening and the USPSTF concludes that the balance of benefits and harm cannot be determined.

Next steps in colorectal cancer screening

There are now two proven methods of reducing mortality from colorectal cancer. These are FOBt performed at least 2-yearly between the ages of 50–74 and once only flexible sigmoidoscopy between the ages 55–64. The interplay between FOBt and flexible sigmoidoscopy has yet to be determined and is particularly important in those countries, such as the UK, where FOBt programmes already exist. In Scotland, people are invited for FOBt screening from 50 so this is a particularly important question.

The Department of Health for England has already announced that flexible sigmoidoscopy screening will be added to the NHS Bowel Cancer Screening Programme with a 5 year roll out period beginning in 2011. It quotes experts as estimating this could save 3,000 lives per year.

Acceptability of the flexible sigmoidoscopy test to the UK population is yet to be determined since only small scale feasibility work has been done. However, the indications are that uptake will be similar to the existing guaiac FOBt programme. It is also suggested that some individuals will accept flexible sigmoidoscopy only and others FOBt only. Thus a combination of the two may increase overall screening coverage in the population. The best test may be the one people actually do.

Further reading

Cancer Research UK. Bowel cancer statistics – Key Facts. http://info .cancerresearchuk.org/cancerstats/types/bowel/ [accessed 10 April 2011].

NHS Bowel Cancer Screening Programme. http://www.cancerscreening.nhs .uk/bowel/about-bowel-cancer-screening.html [accessed 10 April 2011].

Atkin WS, Cuzick J, Northover JM, Whynes DK Prevention of colorectal cancer by once-only sigmoidoscopy. *Lancet*, 1993;**341**:736–740.

Atkin WS, Edwards R, Kralj-Hans I, Wooldrage K, Hart AR, Northover JM, Parkin DM Wardle J, Duffy SW, Cuzick J. UK Flexible Sigmoidoscopy Trial Investigators, Once-only flexible sigmoidoscopy screening in prevention of colorectal cancer: a multicentre randomised controlled trial. *Lancet*, 2010;**375**(9726):1624–1633.

Department of Health. Improving Outcomes: A Strategy for Cancer. London 2011 http://www.dh.gov.uk/en/Publicationsandstatistics/Publications/ PublicationsPolicyAndGuidance/DH_123371 [accessed 10 April 2011].

Hewitson P, Glasziou P, Watson E, Towler B, Irwig L. Cochrane systematic review of colorectal cancer screening using the fecal occult blood test (hemoccult): an update. *Am J Gastroenterol*. 2008;**103**(6):1541–1549.

Johnson CD, Chen MH, Toledano AY, Heiken JP, Dachman A, Kuo MD, Menias CO, Siewert B, Cheema JI, Obregon RG, Fidler JL, Zimmerman P, Horton KM, Coakley K, Iyer RB, Hara AK, Halvorsen RA Jr, Casola G, Yee J, Herman BA, Burgart LJ, Limburg PJ. Accuracy of CT colonography for detection of large adenomas and cancers. *N Engl J Med*. 2008 Sep 18;**359**(12):1207–1217. Erratum in: *N Engl J Med*. 2008; Dec 25;**359**(26): 2853.

Neugut AI, Lebwohl B. Colonoscopy vs sigmoidoscopy screening: getting it right. *JAMA*. 2010;**304**(4):461–462.

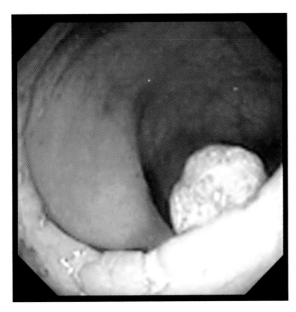

Figure 5.3 Endoscopic view of a bowel polyp.

CHAPTER 6

Decision Support Networks

Matthew Kelly[1], Mark Austin[2] and Sir Michael Brady[3]

[1]Siemens Molecular Imaging, Oxford, UK
[2]IXICO Ltd, London, UK
[3]Department of Radiation Oncology and Biology, Old Road Campus Research Building, Oxford, UK

OVERVIEW

- Multidisciplinary Team (MDT) meetings are pressured, which means important information may be overlooked

- In addition, there has hitherto been almost no IT support for the MDT

- To increase the effectiveness of the role of MDTs an *MDTSuite* tool has been developed and warmly welcomed by clinicians

Introduction

In order to provide the highest level of efficient, standardised, inter-disciplinary patient care, multidisciplinary teams (MDTs) play an increasingly important role in the management of multi-speciality diseases such as cancer. MDT meetings enable a team of clinical specialists (typically a core of surgeons, oncologists, radiologists, pathologists and specialist nurses) to review collectively a patient's clinical information, as well as the decisions taken for the patient at previous MDTs, in order to select the most appropriate management option. The aim is to improve patient management through joined-up thinking and to short-circuit sequential and disconnected analysis by specialists, in which a patient's data are passed in order from Hospital Department to Department. However, these benefits of the MDT require that all the relevant specialities are colocated in a single place, and so it is vital that the meeting proceed as efficiently and effectively as possible.

This implies that the team needs to be presented with all information relevant to the patient management decision in question, avoiding information overload, and that the recommendations made are based on the latest clinical guidelines and evidence, augmented, in cases where the guidelines do not address the current situation, or are inconsistent, by local clinical expertise. Even the most efficient MDTs find these requirements increasingly difficult to satisfy, partly because of the ever-expanding wealth of clinical evidence relating to each of the specialities, but equally because of the increasingly diverse modes of information that may be taken into consideration (e.g. anatomical and functional imaging, genetic studies, immunohistochemistry and new therapeutic options). The sheer quantity of potentially relevant data and evidence, together with the shortage of time, can easily result in information on which a patient management decision is contingent being overlooked, perhaps leading to an inappropriate patient management decision. For example, before the MDT commits to a decision to proceed to CRC surgery, it should take note of whether any previous imaging studies indicated metastatic disease. However, such 'errors of omission' can easily occur in the pressure to discuss all the patients on the MDT list in the limited time available; as many as 30 patients may need to be discussed in a single one-hour meeting, though happily most cases are straightforward and can be processed-rapidly *if the relevant information is to hand and can be presented effectively*. In light of these severe challenges to the MDT, not to mention legal liabilities, it is extraordinary that there continues to be remarkably little, often no, IT support for the MDT meeting (with the exception of the Picture Archiving and Communications System used to retrieve all the radiological images relevant to the patient, from this and possibly previous visits). An IT system has been developed and deployed at our local hospital trust. It has been well received by the CRC MDT.

It is important to understand that the aim of such an IT system is *not* to 'automate' the MDT discussions, or to usurp any of the clinical expertise of the MDT; rather, it is to provide *decision support* and *effective display of the relevant information*.

Fortunately, a number of approaches to providing decision support systems, even in clinical settings, have been developed previously, and we build particularly on the work of Fox and colleagues. Clinical decision support methods generally adopt an approach termed *executable guidelines*, which enables a set of clinical guidelines for a given disease, or class of diseases, to be encoded into a computational system and applied to a specific patient instance. Though details of a number of such prototype systems have been published, only a very few have been applied to routine clinical use. The system developed by our team, *MDT-Suite*, which uses an implementation of argumentation theory, was designed specifically to meet the clinical and practical demands of multidisciplinary care by supporting the MDT meetings for colorectal cancer.

MDTSuite was designed and developed based on extensive observations of CRC MDT meetings and in close collaboration with the

ABC of Colorectal Cancer, Second Edition.
Edited by Annie Young, Richard Hobbs and David Kerr.
© 2011 Blackwell Publishing Ltd. Published 2011 by Blackwell Publishing Ltd.

clinical experts regularly attending these meetings. Specifically, the MDT was supported by:

1 Ensuring all relevant patient data (history, images, histology, etc.) is presented to the MDT when framing a decision, and in cases where such data are not available, ensuring that its potential impact on the clinical decision is appreciated by the MDT.
2 Ensuring the clinical evaluation of the patient information based on the latest clinical evidence and published national clinical guidelines, augmented by local expertise and preferences.
3 Facilitating the capture of a detailed record of each decision taken, including not only the management plan selected, but also the patient data and evidence upon which that selection was contingent, together with a record of those clinicians supporting (or disagreeing with) the decision.

The application

A typical workflow for *MDTSuite* illustrates how the application addresses each of the above considerations.

In preparation for an MDT meeting, data are collected from patient records for all of the patients scheduled for discussion and added to the *system's* database (Figure 6.1). The patient information requested by the system is the set of data with the potential to influence the specific clinical decision being taken for the patient (e.g. the postoperative management decision). These data may be extracted automatically from existing electronic medical records or, when not available, entered manually via an automatically generated input form by the relevant clinical specialist (e.g. radiologist for results of imaging studies).

During the meeting, a patient list (on the left of the screen shot; Figure 6.2) enables the meeting coordinator to sequence through the patients. Once a patient is selected, an automatically generated summary of that patient's information, relevant to the current clinical decision, is displayed (Figure 6.2). This summary integrates information from all of the clinical specialities to provide a rapid overview for each of the MDT members present. Tabs across the top of the page allow the coordinator to step through the additional *pages* for the patient.

The next tab provides a decision history for the patient. This includes the result of all previous discussions by the MDT for the patient, shown on a timeline, along with the reasoning behind the decisions made (Figure 6.3). This reasoning is based on the clinical guidelines encoded in the system and quickly brings the MDT members up-to-date on the patient's stage in the patient journey and obviates the need to recreate the previous discussion and decisions; this would be necessary if only the result of previous decisions were recorded, not the rationale, and MDT membership differed from the previous time the patient was discussed.

The final tab (Figure 6.4) brings up a screen which presents an ordered list of possible treatment options, with those most highly recommended for a given patient given first. The specific component of the encoded guidelines related to each recommendation made (either for or against a particular option; highlighted in green and red, respectively), is presented as an *argument* either *for* or *against* that option. In the example, a circumferential resection margin of less than 1 mm is an argument *against* surgery for the patient. Presenting the guidelines in this way ensures any recommendations made by *the system* are both intuitive and fully transparent. They also relate the relevant patient data to each option, thus aiding the decision-making process of the MDT and providing an efficient mechanism for capturing the full reasoning behind each decision. It should be emphasised that whilst recommendations are made by *the system*, the MDT is free to select any patient management option they choose (or even add a new management option), with the proviso that for non-guideline-recommended options, a reason is provided by the team to ensure a clear record of the decision is maintained. For example, the current emotional state of a patient, along with how they've handled their treatment so far,

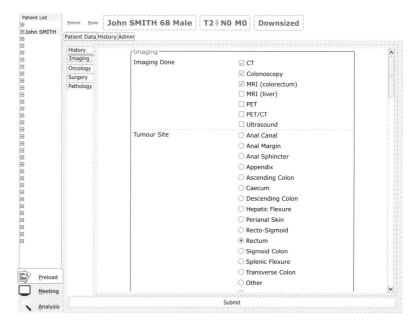

Figure 6.1 Preload screen of *MDTSuite*. This screen is used to enter/acquire the patient information necessary to address the specific clinical question for each patient.

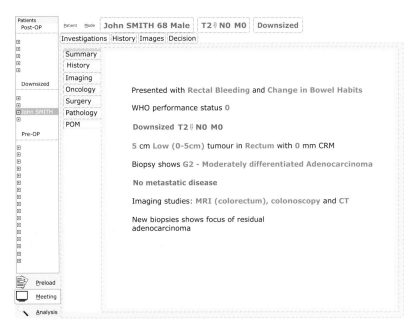

Figure 6.2 Patient summary screen of *MDTSuite*. This screen provides an overview of the clinical information for a given patient, based on the information acquired for both the current MDT meeting along with any previous meetings for that patient.

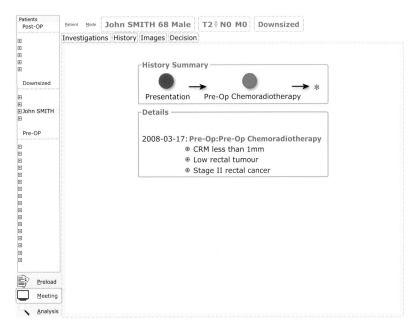

Figure 6.3 Decision history screen of *MDTSuite*. This screen provides a summary of all previous clinical decisions taken for a given patient, along with the guideline-based reasoning relevant to that decision.

can influence the treatment plan significantly; however, this kind of reasoning is difficult to capture in a decision support system.

Alongside the list of treatment options and recommendations is a list of missing data (Figure 6.4). This section highlights any specific pieces of patient data that are not in the system at the time of the meeting, and have the potential to influence the recommendations made by the system for that specific patient (based on the encoded clinical guidelines). In addition, the potential impact of this information on the recommendations made is also provided. For example, for the patient shown in Figure 6.4, if the tumour was known to be tethered (as opposed to mobile; information not in the system at the time of the meeting), then this would be an argument supporting preoperative chemoradiotherapy.

Clinical trial

To assess the suitability of *MDTSuite* for use in the live MDT environment, we have carried out an extensive live trial of the software in our local trust. Over several months, clinical decisions for more than 200 patients were taken using *the system*. In every case, the decision taken along with the underlying reasoning has been successfully recorded.

In practice, the trial required 2 hours a week of researcher time to collect data for the 20–40 patients from their medical records and hospital intranet. A further 4 hours a week was then spent shadowing the radiologist and collaboratively entering the detailed imaging information required for each patient. This collaboration

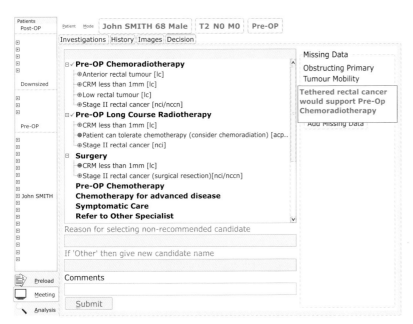

Figure 6.4 Decision screen of *MDTSuite*. This screen provides patient management recommendations based on the clinical guidelines encoded in the application. The MDT is still, however, free to select any option they choose. This screen also highlights any missing data (along with its possible impact) with the potential to influence the recommendations made.

was possible without increasing the workload for the radiologist, and in fact the decision history maintained by the system along with the patient data was frequently a useful resource for the radiologist in building up a picture of each patient, for which they normally rely solely on the radiological reports. It is also worth noting that this researcher preparation time would be minimal if an integrated electronic health record (EHR) system was available. During the meetings, the application was displayed on one of two ceiling-mounted digital projectors, the other of which is used to display radiological and pathological images simultaneously.

Feedback from the trial has been very positive with all clinicians involved describing a benefit to the meetings. A survey of the key members of the CRC MDT highlighted streamlining of the meetings, through case summarisation, integration of multispeciality data and presentation of decision history, as the key benefit of the system. We also believe that as the quality of the encoded guidelines improve, and clinicians become more accustomed to the support they provide, the full value of the decision support engine will become apparent. The results of this trial indicate a changing attitude towards IT and specifically decision support systems in clinical practice. By providing software that not only fits into the existing clinical workflow, but also streamlines and improves it, giving tangible benefit to the clinical users, we were able to gain clinicians' confidence in the system and develop a platform through which the additional benefits of decision support could be delivered. As this trial continues and further improvements are made to the software (e.g. inclusion of an ontological data model), we hope to continue to demonstrate the efficacy of a system like *MDTSuite* in both streamlining the MDT meetings as well as providing an excellent example of a clinically-led decision-making system that may be agreed and utilised nationally.

Further reading

National Cancer Action Team. *The Characteristics of an Effective Multidisciplinary Team* (MDT). NHS, February 2010. http://ncat.nhs.uk/sites/default/files/NCATMDTCharacteristics.pdf [accessed April 20 2011].

Fox J, Rahmanzadeh A. Disseminating medical knowledge: the proforma approach. *Artif Intell Med*, 1998;**14**:157–181.

Sutton D, Fox J. The syntax and semantics of the proforma guide-line modeling language. *Journal of the American Medical Informatics Association*. 2003;**10**:433–443.

CHAPTER 7

Pathology of Colorectal Cancer

Mohammad Ilyas

University of Nottingham, Queen's Medical Centre, Nottingham, UK

OVERVIEW

- The vast majority of malignant tumours in the colon and rectum are adenocarcinomas. These arise as benign precursor lesions known as adenomas which then progress to adenocarcinomas, and this is known as the 'adenoma-carcinoma sequence'

- This 'adenoma-carcinoma sequence' is driven by mutation of genes

- The role of the pathologist is to (i) evaluate biopsy specimens to confirm the diagnosis of adenocarcinoma and (ii) evaluate resection specimens to identify features associated with poor prognosis

- The presence of poor prognostic features may result in the patient receiving adjuvant therapy as well as resection

- Certain gene mutations make tumours non-responsive to some therapies. Identification of these mutations (through molecular diagnostics) allows patients to be managed appropriately

---

Introduction

The pathologist plays a central role in the management of colorectal cancer, from making the initial diagnosis of malignancy to evaluation of the surgical resection specimen. Having covered the Pathways of Carcinogenesis in Chapter 3, the aim of this chapter is to shed light on the role of the pathologist and to clarify the purpose and significance of pathological evaluation of biopsy and resection specimens. In addition, the development of genetic testing of tumours is discussed and future developments in the analysis of tumours are considered.

The development of colorectal cancer

The adenoma-carcinoma sequence

The colon and rectum are lined by glandular epithelium and, although other tissue types are present, the overwhelming majority of malignant colorectal tumours are of epithelial origin. As a general rule, there is a well described pathway of tumour development from benign precursor lesions which progress to malignant adenocarcinomas (see Figure 7.1). As outlined in Chapter 3, this known as the 'adenoma-carcinoma' sequence.

The earliest lesion to develop is an adenoma which will appear as a raised small polyp. Histologically, early adenomas will generally have a 'tubular' appearance reminiscent of normal glandular epithelium but they will also have atypical features (such as nuclear enlargement) which are collectively termed dysplasia. In the early adenomas, the dysplasia will usually be 'low grade' (see Figure 7.2).

As the adenoma (also termed an adenomatous polyp) progresses, it will enlarge and it may develop a stalk or remain sessile. Histologically the appearance will become more complex with some developing a villous appearance whilst others may show a mixed 'tubulo-villous' appearance. The severity of dysplasia will increase and late adenomas will have 'high grade' dysplasia.

Ultimately adenomatous polyps will develop features of malignancy and invade into surrounding tissue at which point it will be regarded as an adenocarcinoma. At the very early stages, a focus of invasion may occur in an adenomatous polyp (called a 'polyp cancer') but eventually surrounding tissues will be destroyed and the cancer may appear as an ulcerated mass. If not removed, the adenocarcinoma may invade through the bowel wall causing perforation and it may metastasise to other sites (usually lymph nodes and liver).

The genetic basis of colorectal cancer

The 'adenoma-carcinoma sequence' is driven by the mutation of important genes. The first mutation is usually of the *APC* gene and this results in the conversion of normal colonic epithelium into an early adenoma. Mutations in other genes (see Figure 7.1) will drive the progression to adenocarcinoma. As the mutations that drive tumour development become identified, it becomes possible to classify tumours on the basis of their genetic changes. Currently colorectal adenocarcinomas are divided into two genetically distinct categories: (a) tumours with chromosomal instability comprising the majority of tumours and (b) tumours with microsatellite instability (MSI) accounting for 10–15% of tumours. These categories are covered in detail in Chapter 3.

ABC of Colorectal Cancer, Second Edition.
Edited by Annie Young, Richard Hobbs and David Kerr.
© 2011 Blackwell Publishing Ltd. Published 2011 by Blackwell Publishing Ltd.

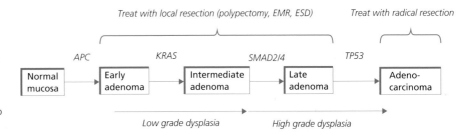

Treat with local resection (polypectomy, EMR, ESD)   Treat with radical resection

Figure 7.1 The adenoma-carcinoma sequence. Tumours arise as benign adenomas which which progress into adenocarcinomas. This is driven by gene mutation (such as *APC, KRAS, SMAD2/4, TP53*). Adenomas can be treated by local or limited resection whilst adenocarcinomas need to be treated by radical resection.

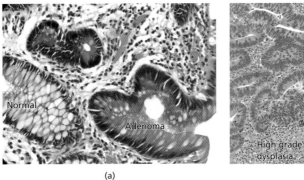
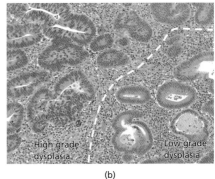

Figure 7.2 (a) Early adenomas are usually tubular adenomas which have low grade dysplasia. (b) One of the features of adenoma progression is increasing severity of dyplasia. In this tumour areas of low and high grade dysplasia are seen within the same tumour.

The role of the pathologist

Evaluation of biopsy specimens

A patient may present to the clinical team because of development of symptoms or through the National Health Service Bowel Cancer Screening Programme (see Chapter 5). This is the starting point of a pathway of management for colorectal tumours (Figure 7.3). An endoscopy will normally be performed and if a suspicious looking lesion is seen (such as an ulcerated mass), then a biopsy will be taken. Whilst malignant lesions are usually obvious at endoscopy, occasional benign lesions may mimic adenocarcinoma and thus histological confirmation of the malignant nature of the lesion is essential. The histological findings will be discussed at the multi-disciplinary team (MDT) meeting (see Chapter 6) and appropriate management will be planned based on histological, clinical and radiological findings. Depending on these findings, a patient may proceed to surgery, receive neo-adjuvant therapy followed by surgery or may be treated palliatively.

Evaluation of local resection specimens

There are a variety of local resection specimens that may be received by the pathologist. Polyps identified during routine colonoscopy may be removed by snare polypectomy, especially if they are seen to have a stalk. Alternatively newer techniques, such as endoscopic mucosal resection (EMR) or endoscopic submucosal dissection (ESD), may be used to remove larger non-malignant polyps. Local resection procedures such as Trans-anal endoscopic microsurgery (TEMS) may occasionally be used in preference to radical resection in the treatment of rectal cancer in cases where the tumour is small and the patient is not fit enough for radical surgery.

A number of key features need to be evaluated in local resection specimens. Firstly, in specimens without a previous biopsy (such

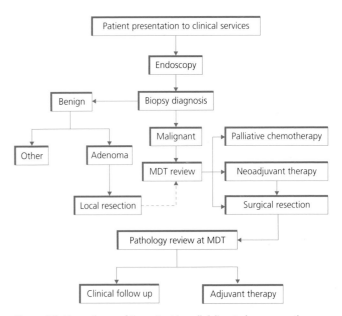

Figure 7.3 The pathway of the patient is well delineated once seen they presents to the clinical team. Pathology of malignant biopsies and radical resection specimens are discussed at the MDT. Local resection specimens for adenomas will only be discussed if malignancy is unexpectedly found.

as snare polypectomy), the neoplastic lesions (i.e. adenomas) need to be distinguished from non-neoplastic lesion (such as a hyperplastic polyp, inflammatory polyp, mucosal prolapse etc.). If it is adenomatous, it will usually be assessed for degree of dysplasia and whether it is completely resected.

If histological examination identifies a polyp cancer (i.e. an adenoma with a focus of invasive malignancy), then other features (such as differentiation, invasion into lymphatics or blood vessels) will also be assessed. Depth of invasion of the tumour will be

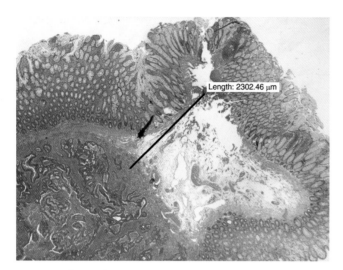

Figure 7.4 If malignancy is unexpectedly found in a polyp resection, the most important evaluation is the distance between tumour and the resection margin. Here the distance is 2 mm and further treatment will probably not be undertaken. A distance of less than 1 mm may require that radical resection be performed.

assessed using the Haggitt staging system (for polyp cancers with stalks) or the Kikuchi system (for sessile polyp cancers). The most important assessment will be of the resection margins. If tumour cells are present at the resection margin or within 1 mm of the resection margin, the tumour will be regarded as incompletely excised and further radical surgery may be required (Figure 7.4).

Evaluation of radical resection specimens
Macroscopic examination

The mainstay of treatment for colorectal adenocarcinoma is radical surgical resection, whereby the segment of bowel containing the tumour is removed together with a segment of mesentery containing lymph nodes which drain the resected segment. On receipt of the resection specimen, the pathologist will firstly examine it macroscopically to look for tumour perforation, the presence of tumour multiplicity and to identify the surgical resection margins. Both the longitudinal margins (i.e. at each end of the specimen) and the circumferential margin (i.e. around the bowel wall) need to be identified and the latter may also be painted to aid histological examination (Figure 7.5). For rectal tumours, the quality of the mesorectal fascia will also be assessed as an indicator of the quality of surgery and the likelihood of complete resection.

It is not possible to histologically examine a resection specimen in its entirety, so the pathologist will usually take some samples of the tumour and will try to recover as many lymph nodes from the mesentery as possible. The purpose of pathological evaluation is to (a) stage the disease and (b) ascertain the presence of other features indicating poor prognosis (Tables 7.1 and 7.2, Figure 7.6).

Tumour staging

The stage of a tumour – whether clinical or pathological – is basically a description of the spread of that tumour. This informs on prognosis since the more advanced the stage of a tumour (i.e. the

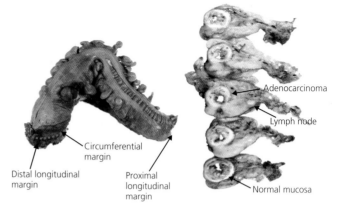

Figure 7.5 Resection specimens will usually be examined macroscopically to identify the surgical resection margins (proximal, distal and circumferential). The specimens will sliced and samples taken of the tumour and the lymph nodes.

Table 7.1 Tumour staging in colorectal cancer.

TNM stage	Dukes' stage	Prognosis
T1N0 M0 T2N0 M0	Duke's A	5 year survival >90%
T3N0M0 T4N0M0	Duke's B	5 year survival 70–85% 5 year survival 55–65%
Any T, N1M0	Dukes' C (C1 if apical node negative)	5 year survival 45–55%
Any T, N2M0	(C2 if apical node positive)	5 year survival 20–30%
any T, any N, M1	Duke's D	5 year survival <5%

Tumour staging is a description of cancer spread and gives an indication of prognosis. Two different staging systems are commonly used – the TNM staging and Dukes' staging – although both can be correlated with each other. T1 = invasion into submucosa; T2 = invasion into muscularis propria; T3 = invasion through the muscularis propria; T4 = invasion through the serosa or into adjacent organs. N1 = metastasis to three or less nodes; N2 = metastasis to more than three nodes. M1 = metastasis to any distant site.

greater the tumour spread) the poorer the prognosis. In the UK, two main staging systems are used for colorectal cancers: the Dukes' system and the TNM (Tumour, Nodes, Metastasis) system (Table 7.1). The latter system individually classifies local spread (the T-stage), lymph node spread (the N-stage) and distant metastasis (the M-stage) whilst the Dukes' system also assesses these features but combines them together in the final stage. Both systems evaluate local spread in relation to local anatomical landmarks but do not include the size of the tumour.

In some instances, especially with rectal cancer, the patient may have received neoadjuvant therapy before surgery. In these cases the T-stage may be prefixed with the letter 'y' to indicate that this therapy has been administered. The effect of neoadjuvant therapy may be to cause regression of the tumour with fibrous scar tissue replacing the tumour tissue. In these cases the degree of regression may be also be evaluated using the Mandard grading system.

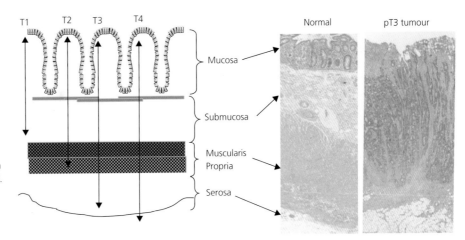

Figure 7.6 The normal colon has a structure comprising mucosa, submucosa, muscularis propria and serosa/adventitia (shown in cartoon form on the left and histologically in the centre). The pathological T stage is a measurement of local invasion in relation to these anatomical structures and a pT3 tumour (i.e. invasion into the serosa) is shown on the right.

Table 7.2 Prognostic features in colorectal cancer.

Poor prognostic features in colorectal cancer	Good prognostic features in colorectal cancer
pT4 (tumour perforation, breaching of serosal surface, invasion into surrounding organs)*	Microsatellite instability
Extramural vascular invasion*	Dense intra-tumoural lymphocytes
Poor differentiation (i.e. Grade 3)*	Pushing tumour edge
Involvement of resection margin*	
Recovery of small number of lymph nodes*	
Infiltrative tumour edge and tumour budding	
Peri-neural invasion	

Certain features of a tumour are indicative of a poor prognosis and may result in adjuvant chemotherapy being administered even in the absence of lymph node metastasis. These features are listed here and those marked with an asterisk are part of the minimum data set. The right hand column shows features which have been associated with good prognosis.

Poor prognostic features

As well as tumour stage, other features of colorectal tumours have been identified which seem to be associated with a poor prognosis (Table 7.2). If these features are identified after histological examination, the patient may be considered for adjuvant chemotherapy. In addition, the surgical margins will be assessed histologically. As with polyp cancers, the margin will be deemed involved by tumour (with the implication that resection is incomplete) if tumour cells are present either at the resection margin or within 1 mm of the resection margin. If there is margin involvement, then further therapy (such as radiotherapy) may be considered.

The Royal College of Pathologists in the UK has produced a minimum data set which should be completed for every resection specimen. The minimum data set contains information on tumour stage, the presence of poor prognostic features and the completeness of resection. After a resection specimen has been evaluated, the findings will be discussed at the MDT and further decisions will be made on the management of the patient. As a general rule, all tumours with metastasis to lymph nodes (or other more distant sites) will receive adjuvant chemotherapy. Tumours may receive adjuvant chemotherapy if one of the poor prognostic features is present even in the absence of nodal metastasis.

Liver metastases

It has been shown that partial hepatectomy for resection of discrete metastatic deposits in the liver can improve patient outcome. Some of the newer biological therapies (see predictive testing) can induce regression in tumour deposits thereby allowing previously unresectable metastases to be resected. It is thus not uncommon now for hepatic tumour deposits to be treated with surgical resection. Depending on the timing of the surgery, the histological appearances will vary. Thus if the liver resection is performed after chemotherapy, then the hepatectomy specimen may show tumour regression similar to that seen after neoadjuvant therapy. If partial hepatectomy is undertaken synchronously with surgery for the primary tumour, the specimen will not show regression of the tumour. Pathological evaluation of partial hepatectomy specimens is primarily to assess the surgical margins and ensure that resection is complete.

Adjunctive tests

For histological evaluation, sections taken from pathology specimens are usually stained with Haematoxylin and Eosin (H&E). In the vast majority of instances this is sufficient to make the diagnosis and to evaluate prognostic features. In certain situations, however, supplementary tests are required to facilitate the diagnostic process. Such situations include (a) when there is doubt about the origin of the primary tumour (i.e. it is uncertain whether the tumour is a primary colorectal adenocarcinoma or whether it is an adenocarcinoma which has arisen at another site but is involving the colon/rectum), (b) when there is a liver metastasis of uncertain origin, (c) when there is uncertainty about vascular invasion, (d) when the primary tumour is not of epithelial origin and (e) when there is a need to test for mismatch repair proteins (see below). The supplementary tests include *histochemistry* whereby special

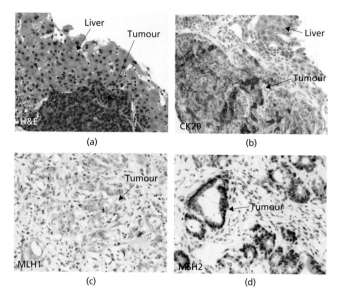

Figure 7.7 (a & b) show how special tests such as immunohistochemistry can be used to identify the origin of a tumour metastasis. (a) shows the H&E section of a tumour deposit in the liver and (b) shows that expression of CK20 in the tumour confirms the origin as colorectal. (c & d) show a tumour with microsatellite instability due to loss of MLH1. Immunohistochemistry has been used to show that tumours cells do not show MLH1 expression whilst MSH2 expression is unaffected.

stains are applied to tissue sections to identify specific cell or tissue types and *immunohistochemistry* whereby monoclonal antibodies are applied to tissue sections to identify specific molecules expressed by cells (Figure 7.7). These are used to help to resolve the diagnostic difficulties.

Molecular diagnostics

Molecular diagnostics can be viewed as the testing of tumour derived DNA, RNA or protein for the purpose of facilitating diagnosis or management decisions. Currently there are two main uses for molecular diagnostics in the management of colorectal cancer.

Microsatellite instability and chromosomal instability

Colorectal adenocarcinomas can be divided into at least two distinct genetic categories – tumours with microsatellite instability (MSI) and tumours with chromosomal instability, also discussed in Chapter 3. Tumours with MSI comprise around 10–15% of colorectal adenocarcinomas and tend to have a different spectrum of mutations to those found in tumours with chromosomal instability. These genetic differences are reflected in differences in both histological appearance and tumour biology. Tumours with MSI tend to be located in the right colon; histologically they are often poorly differentiated, mucinous and associated with a dense lymphocytic infiltrate. Tumours with MSI are usually less advanced than tumours with chromosomal instability and tend to have a

better overall prognosis. In addition, there is evidence that tumours with MSI may be less responsive to 5-Fluorouracil (which is the main chemotherapeutic agent currently used in colorectal cancer).

MSI arises due to loss of any one of four mismatch repair genes. In the majority of cases of sporadic cancer with MSI, there is loss of *MLH1* function although loss of *MSH2; MSH6* and *PMS2* would also cause MSI. Testing for MSI can be done by immunohistochemistry for expression of the mismatch repair proteins (Figure 7.7). Alternatively, testing can be done using the Polymerase Chain Reaction (PCR) with a panel of five markers known as the Bethesda panel. The PCR is performed on DNA and thus, for this test, DNA needs to be extracted from the tumour.

Predictive testing

In recent years a number of new therapies have been developed for the treatment of cancer. Amongst these, the most conspicuous are the biological therapies (also known as 'biologics') which consist of monoclonal antibodies targeted against certain molecules which are present on tumour cells. The best known biologic is Herceptin, which targets the *c-ErbB2* gene and is used in the treatment of breast cancer. For the treatment of colorectal cancer, biologics have been developed which target the Epidermal Growth Factor Receptor (EGFR). Some tumours show dramatic response to these biologics whilst other tumours, despite the expression of EGFR, remain unresponsive. It has become apparent that mutation of the *KRAS* gene renders colorectal tumours non-responsive to anti-EGFR therapies. A tumour can be therefore tested for the presence of *KRAS* mutation in order to 'predict' whether it is likely to respond before commencing treatment with anti-EGFR biologics. This is known as predictive testing and, given the potential side effects and financial costs of such treatments, it is essential that predictive testing is performed when a known test is available.

Future perspectives

Without doubt the most significant developments in the next decade will be in the field of molecular diagnostics. The rapid development of technologies means that it is now feasible that, in the near future, every single colorectal cancer will undergo complete sequencing of its DNA to identify all the mutations that are present within the tumour. This will drive classification of tumours based on the mutation profile of tumours. Once the significance of the mutations is completely understood, it will be possible to tailor a bespoke therapeutic regime for each individual tumour. Appropriate targeting of tumours may even change first line treatment from surgery to chemotherapy. Despite this, the basic morphological evaluation of the specimen will still be necessary since molecular diagnostics may not easily distinguish early adenocarcinoma from advanced adenoma nor will it indicate whether resection margins are clear. The role of the pathologist will inevitably change to one of integrating the molecular diagnostics with the 'standard' pathology in order to provide the best data to MDT for planning management of the patient.

CHAPTER 8

Imaging of Colorectal Cancer

Andrew Slater

John Radcliffe Hospital, Oxford, UK

OVERVIEW

- Diagnosis of colorectal cancer can be by Colonoscopy or CT Colonography, which have equal sensitivity. Minimal preparation CT of the Colon is a less accurate test that is very easy to tolerate

- Staging of colorectal cancer is by CT of the whole body. MRI is also used to stage rectal cancer, and endoscopic ultrasound is useful for early rectal tumours. MRI of the liver and PET/CT are not used routinely, but are helpful in staging complex cases

- Follow up of metastatic disease, and surveillance in cured patients is usually carried out with CT scanning

- Liver metastases can be treated successfully with Radiofrequency ablation as a percutaneous procedure

- Bowel obstruction from colon cancer can be treated successfully with self-expanding metal stents placed endoluminally under radiological guidance

---

Diagnosis of colorectal cancer

Optical colonoscopy (OC) and Computed Tomography Colonography (CTC) have equivalent very high sensitivities for detecting colorectal cancer of around 98%. The terms Virtual Colonoscopy and CT pneumocolon are synonymous with CTC. OC requires full laxative bowel preparation and sedation. It is expensive, occasionally causes bowel perforation, but has the advantage of immediate biopsy of detected lesions and can detect non-malignant process such as colitis.

There has recently been a UK National Patient Safety Agency (NPSA) initiative regarding laxative bowel preparation (Picolax, Citrafleet, Fleet Phospho-Soda, Klean Prep, Moviprep). This was stimulated by reported incidents of harm from use of these drugs, including one death. It is no longer acceptable for UK Radiology departments to send patients laxative bowel preparation in the post based upon the very limited clinical information usually available on a radiology request card. In future all requests for examinations that use laxative bowel preparation (Colonoscopy, CT Colonography

and Barium Enema) must state explicitly that the patient is safe to take these medicines, for example stating 'patient fit for laxative bowel prep'.

Information regarding cautions and contraindications to these drugs is available in the British National Formulary (BNF), but the main risks are of bowel perforation in patients with acute diverticulitis, and electrolyte imbalance in patients who are also taking diuretic medication or have renal impairment. Information regarding safe use of laxatives is provided for patients when these drugs are dispensed, and referring clinicians are asked to emphasise to patients the importance of following these instructions.

CTC was first described using laxative bowel preparation, but techniques have been developed that use oral contrast agents for 24–48 hours and a modified diet instead. This technique is called faecal tagging; faecal material that remains in the colon will be 'tagged' with oral contrast and so can easily be distinguished from pathology (Figure 8.1). The NPSA regulations described above do not apply to this type of preparation. When the patient attends for the CT scan, a small tube is placed in the back passage and CO_2 is insufflated until the colon is distended. CO_2 is absorbed much more rapidly by the bowel than air, and so greatly reduces

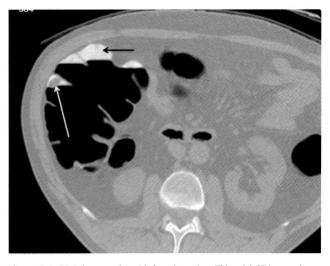

Figure 8.1 CT Colonography with faecal tagging. This axial CT image shows some residual faecal fluid within the colon, but this is high attenuation due to the tagging material (black arrow). A small polyp can be easily distinguished from this fluid (white arrow).

ABC of Colorectal Cancer, Second Edition.
Edited by Annie Young, Richard Hobbs and David Kerr.
© 2011 Blackwell Publishing Ltd. Published 2011 by Blackwell Publishing Ltd.

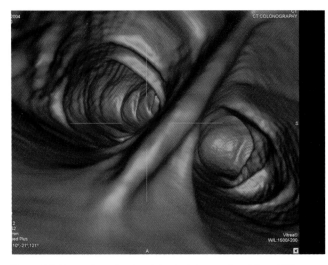

Figure 8.2 Three-dimensional endoluminal view produced from CTC, mimicking an endoscopic view.

discomfort after the procedure. Patients will usually be scanned twice, prone and supine. Any faecal residue remaining within the colon will move with gravity between the two scans, enabling it to be distinguished from tumours and polyps. Three-dimensional images of the gas-distended colon can be made using sophisticated software (Figure 8.2).

A modified form of this examination is Minimal Preparation CT of the Colon (MPCT Colon). Patients take small amounts of oral contrast agent with food for 48 hours before the examination. No diet modification or gas insufflation is used (Figure 8.3). This test is less sensitive for cancer (around 95%), but is very easy to tolerate. CT scanning uses a moderate amount of radiation and should therefore be avoided in young people, in whom OC is preferred. CTC has great benefit as a cheap, accurate and safe test for colorectal cancer, and can be used without laxatives. MPCT Colon

is generally reserved for the frail elderly. The barium enema is no longer considered sensitive enough at detecting cancer to be used.

Staging of colorectal cancer

Colon cancer is staged by CT of the chest, abdomen and pelvis. Intravenous contrast is used, but bowel preparation is not required. The examination usually takes 15 minutes or less with the actual scan time being under a minute. Staging is by the TNM system. CT cannot distinguish between T1 and T2, and is poor at nodal staging unless the nodes are grossly enlarged. CT is good at detecting T4 involvement of adjacent organs (Figure 8.4), but is poor at detecting T4 involvement to the peritoneum.

CT is generally accurate at detecting metastases, although MRI of the liver is more accurate for detecting metastases to this organ. MRI

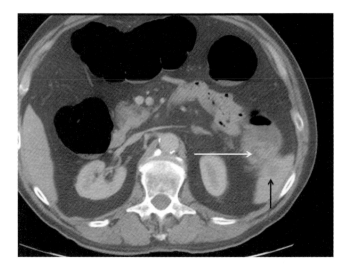

Figure 8.4 Axial CT image of a tumour of the splenic flexure (white arrow). This abuts the spleen, and low attenuation within the spleen indicates tumour invasion (black arrow), making this T4.

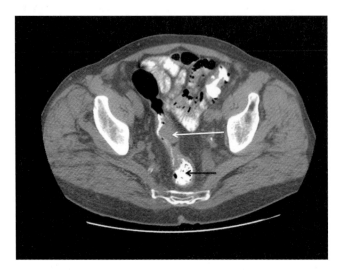

Figure 8.3 MPCT Colon. This axial CT image shows how high attenuation tagged faeces (black arrow) can easily be distinguished from a small polypoid tumour (white arrow). Note that the colon is not distended with gas, and the faecal material is more solid than in Figure 8.1.

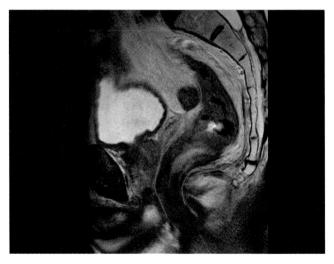

Figure 8.5 A sagittal MRI scan of the pelvis. The rectum fills the posterior pelvis. An embryological remnant, the mesorectal fascia surrounds the rectum and is outlined in red. This is the standard surgical resection plane.

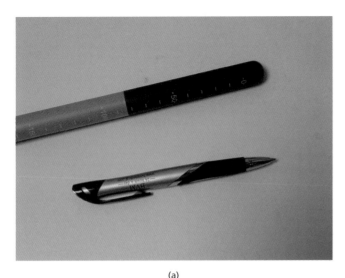

(a)

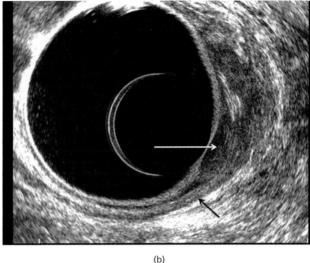

(b)

Figure 8.6 (a) A transrectal ultrasound probe with a pen for size comparison. A water-filled balloon is usually placed over then end of this probe, to enable contact with the rectal wall. (b) An endoluminal ultrasound image of the rectum. The central black part of the image represents the probe and water within the balloon. The white arrow demonstrates a small rectal polyp. Two black lines are seen in the normal rectal wall. The outer one (black arrow) is the muscularis propria.

is often used in combination with CT for indeterminate lesions. MRI scanning generally takes 30 minutes, and would usually use a Gadolinium injection as a contrast agent.

Patients with mobile metal within their bodies usually cannot enter an MRI scanner, although some modern pacemakers are reported to be MRI compatible. Ultrasound of the liver is cheap and radiation free, but is unfortunately not reliable at excluding metastases.

MRI is used for local staging of rectal cancer to determine the relationship of the tumour to the standard surgical resection plane or circumferential resection margin (CRM). This is a thin layer of fibrous tissue around the perirectal fat called the mesorectal fascia (MRF) (Figure 8.5). Tumours which are close to this plane would be considered for downsizing chemoradiotherapy before surgery, to reduce the risk of local recurrence.

Transrectal ultrasound can be used to accurately T stage early rectal tumours. An ultrasound probe is placed within the rectum very close to the tumour (Figure 8.6). It can distinguish between T1, 2 and 3. However it does not have sufficient depth to assess the CRM, and can only assess lymph nodes that are close to the tumour. This can help select those patients in whom Transanal Endoscopic Microsurgery (TEM) is considered as an alternative to standard proctectomy. This technique is uncomfortable, but is generally no worse than a flexible sigmoidoscopy.

Positron emission tomography (PET/CT) is a combination modality that is highly accurate for the detection of metastatic disease, although it has a high radiation burden and is expensive. It is not routinely used for staging, but would be considered before surgery for resection or for problem solving. Patients are injected with deoxyglucose labelled with radioactive 18Fluorine (FDG). This is taken up avidly by malignant cells, and its presence is detected when it decays to produce positrons. A CT scanner is sited adjacent to the positron detectors and provides anatomical

detail. Thus a hybrid image can be produced of a CT scan with FDG activity overlaid on a colour scale (Figure 8.7). FDG normally shows avid uptake in the brain and heart muscle. It is excreted in the urine, and so high activity is seen in the kidney, ureters and bladder. FDG is also taken up by active muscles, so patients are asked to sit quietly for 45–90 minutes between the injection and commencement of scanning. A pitfall is that areas of inflammation can often be FDG avid as well. After a PET/CT patients will remain radioactive for several hours, and are advised to avoid contact with children and pregnant women for the rest of the day.

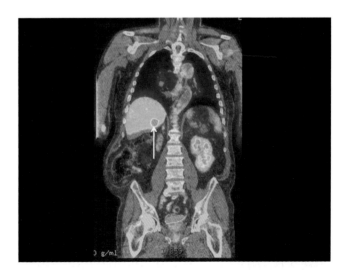

Figure 8.7 Coronal hybrid PET/CT image. A CT image has been overlaid with a colour map of FDG uptake, with red indicating the greatest uptake. A liver metastasis (white arrow) shows increased FDG activity. Note the normal high activity in the left kidney (right kidney not seen on this image) and bladder due to urinary excretion of FDG.

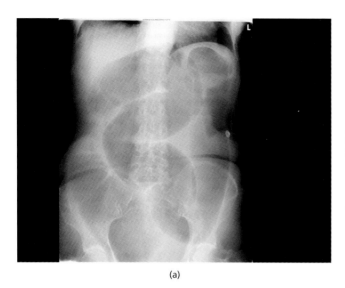

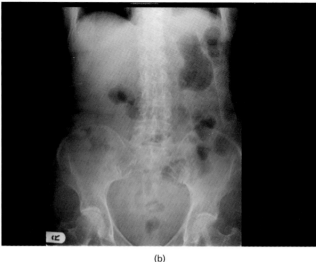

(a)   (b)

Figure 8.8 (a) Plain abdominal x-ray shows gross gaseous dilatation of the colon representing large bowel obstruction due to a descending colon cancer. (b) A subsequent image after endoluminal placement of a metal stent shows resolution of the bowel obstruction.

Stenting of obstructing tumours

A minority of colorectal tumours present with acute large bowel obstruction. CT is the best investigation for patients with large bowel obstruction, and can usually make the diagnosis, although such tumours are frequently small. Current practice is to place a self-expanding metal stent in the tumour under x-ray guidance to relieve the bowel obstruction (Figure 8.8). Definitive surgery can then be planned at a later date. Complications of stents include migration and perforation. Migration of the stent describes a stent moving distal to the tumour, so patients then develop bowel obstruction again. Perforation occurs when the metal of the stent erodes through the tumour, and will present in the same way as any other bowel perforation (Figure 8.9). This can be treated by placement of a second, covered stent, or more commonly by

surgical resection. A covered stent has a plastic coating over the wire mesh.

Follow-up of metastatic disease

CT is the mainstay of follow-up of metastatic colorectal disease to monitor the response to chemotherapy. Radiofrequency ablation (RFA) of liver metastases involves placing a probe within the metastasis percutaneously under CT guidance, and applying a radiofrequency current that causes necrosis in the tumour cells. This is done under general anaesthetic. It is now commonly used in combination with conventional hepatic surgery, and both can be curative if this is the only site of metastatic disease. Patients with advanced metastatic disease can develop bowel obstruction from growth of the primary tumour. This can be treated with a radiologically placed self-expanding metal stent as described above, and this can obviate the need for surgery at all.

Surveillance

It is generally agreed that there is benefit to using imaging to look for recurrent disease in patients thought to have been cured of colorectal cancer. The main advantage is in detection of liver metastases, which may be treated with curative intent by surgical excision or by RFA. There is no consensus upon which scans to use and their timing, but generally a CT scan of the abdomen and pelvis at one year after surgery is used. The CT may also include the chest, and can be combined with a colon preparation to look for new colon tumours.

Further reading

Herbertson RA, Scarsbrook AF, Lee ST, Tebbutt N, Scott AM. Established, emerging and future roles of PET/CT in the management of

Figure 8.9 Photograph of a surgically resected segment of colon containing stented tumour. The end of the forceps mark the point where the metal stent has eroded through the colon wall, causing bowel perforation.

colorectal cancer. *Clin Radiol*. 2009 Mar;**64**(3):225–237. Epub 2008, Oct 23.

Iannaccone R, Laghi A, Catalano C, Mangiapane F, Lamazza A, Schillaci A, Sinibaldi G, Murakami T, Sammartino P, Hori M, Piacentini F, Nofroni I, Stipa V, Passariello R. Computed tomographic colonography without cathartic preparation for the detection of colorectal polyps. *Gastroenterology* 2004 Nov;**127**(5):1300–1311.

Rockey DC. Computed tomographic colonography: current perspectives and future directions. *Gastroenterology* 2009 Jul;**137**(1):7–14. Epub 2009 May 18.

The Royal College of Radiologists, *Consensus Guidelines for the Prescription and Administration of Oral Bowel Cleansing Agents* http://www.rcr.ac.uk/publications.aspx?PageID=310&PublicationID=309 [accessed 10 April 2011].

CHAPTER 9

The Role of Primary Care

Sue Wilson[1] and Richard Hobbs[2]

[1]University of Birmingham, Birmingham, UK
[2]Department of Primary Care Health Sciences, University of Oxford, UK

OVERVIEW

Primary care has an important but often under-utilised role in colorectal cancer in:

- Heath promotion
- Advice concerning genetic risk
- Encouraging participation in screening
- Early recognition of symptoms that warrant further investigation

Key functions after diagnosis include:

- Encompassing the coordination of continuity of care
- Providing ongoing support for patients, carers and families
- Providing or coordinating palliative care to patients
- Supporting families and carers, through dying and provision of bereavement care

---

Box 9.1 **Initiatives to increase earlier diagnosis of colorectal cancer**

- population-based screening
- increasing public awareness of relevant symptoms
- reducing the delay between onset of symptoms
- first presentation
- increasing awareness of relevant ('red flag') symptoms
- identifying methods to better differentiate between cases requiring routine or urgent referral
- improving the accuracy of diagnostic interventions

Introduction

Colorectal cancer is the second most common cancer in England. Despite improvements in survival during the last decade, the 5-year survival rate remains at less than 50%. Earlier diagnosis of colorectal cancer is associated with improved survival. Compared to other Western European countries, UK patients present with more advanced disease and consequently have poorer survival. Men, older people and socially deprived groups are more likely to present late. The deprivation gap in survival for many cancers, including colorectal cancer, has actually been widening; this may be due to a combination of treatment factors, poorer outcome after surgery, poorer general health and lower uptake of screening (see Chapter 5). In addition to improved survival, the benefits of earlier diagnosis include an improved quality of life and reduced treatment costs. Nevertheless, many patients do not present early and less than 15% of tumours are localised at the time of diagnosis. Most colorectal cancers first present to primary care, therefore, GPs have a key role in improving the early detection of patients who have symptoms (Box 9.1).

General practitioners not only have a key role in the identification of suspected new cancers and arranging appropriate referral. Subsequent to primary treatment, they also are involved in the provision of supportive care and in ensuring that care is appropriately coordinated.

Almost 1 million people visit their GP every day in the UK. The average GP sees 40 to 50 patients a day, but will only see one new case of colorectal cancer each year. Many of the symptoms of colorectal cancer are common and non-specific including rectal bleeding, altered bowel habit, abdominal pain, iron deficiency anaemia or tiredness. Distinguishing colorectal cancer from other more common disorders is a significant challenge.

Primary care has a significant contribution to make in all stages of the cancer journey (Figure 9.1), particularly in the early diagnosis of the condition and in encouraging participation in the NHS Bowel Cancer Screening Programme (NHS BCSP – Chapter 5), but also in monitoring patients after curative procedures and in palliation of symptoms in those with established disease.

Early diagnosis and referral guidelines

Early diagnosis of colorectal cancer is essential in view of the stage related prognosis. Five-year survival rates for colorectal cancer are significantly correlated with affluence; this is attributed to earlier stage at presentation and hence earlier resection among those from affluent backgrounds. Survival differentials may be exacerbated by lower screening uptake in deprived areas. There is a need to reduce inequalities in health. Significant delays to

---

ABC of Colorectal Cancer, Second Edition.
Edited by Annie Young, Richard Hobbs and David Kerr.
© 2011 Blackwell Publishing Ltd. Published 2011 by Blackwell Publishing Ltd.

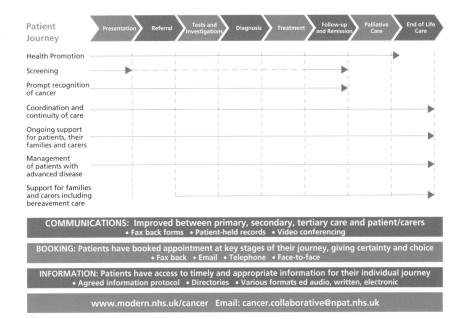

Figure 9.1 The patient journey. Source: *Cancer in Primary Care, A Guide to Good Practice*, NHS Modernisation Agency 2004.

diagnosis/treatment observed in the 1990s led to the NHS Cancer Plan and considerable progress has been made. However, there is still scope for improvement and in Cancer Reform Strategy, 'Improving Outcomes: A Strategy for Cancer' in 2011 the priority action area was earlier diagnosis of cancer including: improving and expanding screening, public awareness of signs and symptoms and a better understanding of the nature and extent of delays in cancer diagnosis.

Three potential levels of delay occur in the diagnosis of the disease: delay by the patient in presenting to the general practitioner; delay in referral by the general practitioner to a specialist; and delay by the hospital in either establishing the diagnosis or starting treatment. A recent systematic review identified evidence for factors associated with pre-hospital delay (Box 9.2).

Box 9.2 **Factors associated with pre-hospital delay in diagnosis**

Patient:

- the type of symptom (altered bowel habit)
- non-recognition of symptom seriousness
- denial of symptom
- fear
- lower education
- living alone
- rural locations

Physician:

- lack of continuity of care
- failure to examine/investigate
- initial misdiagnosis
- inaccurate/inadequate tests
- patient's social class
- younger age

rectal cancer
non-use of referral guidelines

Source: Adapted from Mitchell 2007

Patients presenting with symptoms

Most patients developing colorectal cancer will eventually present with symptoms, although many large bowel symptoms are common and non-specific and often present late. Rectal bleeding, for example, affects up to 20% of the general population and in most cases, cancer is not the cause. Other lower gastrointestinal symptoms that are experienced relatively frequently by people in the community include change in bowel habit, abdominal pain, mucus and tenesmus. Individual symptoms are poor predictors of cancer. The National Institute for Clinical Excellence (NICE) clinical guideline on referral for suspected cancer make specific recommendations about which patients should be urgently referred – within two weeks – for further investigation in the NHS (NICE 2005) (Figure 9.2). The guidelines also indicate which symptoms are highly unlikely to be caused by colorectal cancer.

Blood mixed with or on the stool and change in bowel habit are the most consistent predictors of colorectal cancer. The combination of age, bleeding mixed with or on the stool and change in bowel habit are indications for an urgent referral for further investigation. Iron deficiency anaemia can be the presenting sign of colorectal cancer, although this diagnosis is not the most frequent cause of anaemia. Suggestive findings on rectal examination are a strong predictor of the presence of cancer. Clinical examination may show a definite right sided abdominal mass or definite rectal mass.

The risk of colorectal cancer in young people is low (99% occur in people aged over 40 years and 85% in those aged over 60). In patients aged under 40, therefore, initial management will depend on whether they have a family history of colorectal cancer – namely, a first degree relative (brother, sister, parent or child) with colorectal cancer presenting below the age of 55, or two or more affected second degree relatives. Patients aged under 40 presenting with alarm symptoms and a family history of the disease should also be urgently referred for further investigation. In the absence of a family history of the disease, younger patients with a negative physical examination, including a digital rectal examination, can be initially treated symptomatically. If symptoms persist, however, patients should be considered for further investigation.

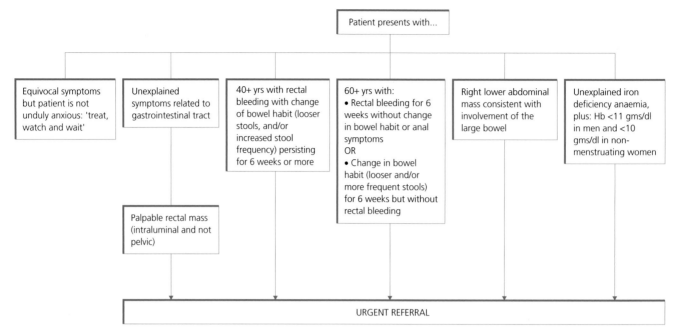

Figure 9.2 Urgent referral algorithm. Source: NICE (2005) Referral Guidelines for Suspected Cancer in Adults and Children. Clinical guideline 27. National Institute for Health and Clinical Excellence. www.nice.org.uk June 2005.

In patients suspected of having colorectal cancer, referral should be indicated as urgent (with an appointment expected within two weeks); the referral letter should include any relevant family history and details about symptoms and risk factors. An increasing number of general practitioners will have direct access to investigations, often via a rapid access rectal bleeding clinic. The usual investigations needed will be flexible sigmoidoscopy or barium enema studies.

Patients with genetic predisposition

All patients registering with a practice for the first time should provide details of their medical history. Patients with a history of familial adenomatous polyposis (see Chapter 4) should be referred for DNA testing before the age of 15. Patients with a positive result should enter a programme of regular surveillance by flexible sigmoidoscopy.

The second common genetic predisposition to colorectal cancer is hereditary non-polyposis colon cancer (HNPCC). This condition should be suspected in patients describing three or more cases of colorectal cancer (or adenocarcinoma of the uterus) within their family. Such patients should be referred for endoscopic screening at the age of 25. Genetic testing for this condition may be possible if DNA is available from an affected relative. Molecular tumour studies may help identify which gene and families should be investigated further. For details on clinical management, see Chapter 4.

Population screening in primary care

Primary care has a key role in supporting evidence-based lifestyle changes (Chapter 2) that could prevent the occurrence of cancer, promoting screening and initiating earlier investigation and diagnosis. Benefits of earlier diagnosis include improved survival and quality of life and reduced treatment costs.

The NHS BCSP is covered comprehensively in Chapter 5. This has been a success; however, primary care clinicians are concerned that uptake rates for the NHSBCSP are significantly lower in men, younger people, those from deprived areas and those from the Indian sub-continent. An added concern is that it appears that uptake is falling in rounds subsequent to the prevalent round.

Managing patients with established disease

After confirmation of diagnosis, the role of the primary care team revolves around providing advice and support, possibly monitoring for recurrence, and palliative care. Some general practices are involved with home based chemotherapy, usually coordinated by specialist outreach nurses.

In the United Kingdom primary care does not yet have a formal role in monitoring for disease recurrence after curative treatments. Data on this option are relatively limited but do suggest that such surveillance could be safely conducted in primary care (see Chapter 16). Ideally, this monitoring should be accompanied by adequate infrastructure and training in primary care, with good liaison between the practice and secondary (or tertiary) care.

Limited evidence from other types of shared care indicate that certain factors are likely to improve outcomes: structured and planned discharge policies; the use of shared (preferably patient held) cards that document patient information (disease progress and drug treatments, as a minimum); locally agreed guidelines specifying the appropriate follow up and delineating responsibilities; and access to rapid referral clinics. As with follow up in all chronic diseases, good communication between doctors and their patients and their families results in better quality of care.

Where appropriate, the doctor should also counsel patients on any possible familial risk and the need for genetic counselling of relatives. The primary care doctor may also advise patients with diagnosed colorectal cancer about practical considerations, including access to social security benefits. In the United Kingdom eligibility for attendance allowance may be immediately available in the exceptional circumstance of cancer with a short terminal prognosis of less than six months.

For some patients, especially those with rectal tumours, the diagnosis of cancer is also accompanied by the necessity for either colostomy or ileostomy. Such patients will often require further specialised support, and liaison between the primary care team and specialist stoma nurses is important (see Chapter 15).

As colorectal cancer is the sixth most common cause of mortality in the United Kingdom, a general practitioner will on average care for a patient dying from colorectal cancer every 18 months. As the disease progresses, management will shift towards palliative care. Ideally, this would be delivered jointly by the primary care team and specialist palliative care services, such as those based at a hospice or provided by specialist palliative care nurses. Few data exist to guide on the most effective models for palliative care in colorectal cancer. However, non-randomised studies have shown high satisfaction among patients when they are kept fully involved in understanding the progression of their disease and their treatment options, when shared care cards are used, and when home care teams are provided. Complex symptomatic care in some cases can be enhanced by admission to a specialist unit when specialist care is not available or manageable at home.

A shared (between healthcare sectors) end of life pathway is in use in most parts of the UK. The patient and carer preference for where the patient wishes to die should be documented and updated as part of the pathway and primary care clinicians, as part of the palliative care team, will realise those wishes where at all possible.

Conclusion

Whilst it was often perceived that the key role of primary care was limited to a gatekeeper function, ensuring appropriate cases are referred for secondary care investigation, it is now acknowledged that it has a significant contribution to make in all stages of the cancer pathway. Indeed with the governmental changes in England only, primary care will lead the commissioning and provision of healthcare. Heath promotion, advice concerning genetic risk and encouraging participation in screening will assist in the prevention of disease and in early diagnosis. Early recognition of symptoms that warrant further investigation remains an important part of the primary care role. There are also key functions after diagnosis: encompassing the coordination of continuity of care; providing ongoing support for patients, carers and families; providing palliative care to patients; and supporting families and carers, including the provision of bereavement care. At all these stages, primary care plays an important role not only in the management of disease but also in the provision of information to assist in decision making.

Further reading

Coleman MP, Rachet B, Woods LM, Mitry E, Riga M, Cooper N, Quinn MJ, Brenner H, Estève J. Trends and socioeconomic inequalities in cancer survival in England and Wales up to 2001. *Br J Cancer* 2004;**90**: 1367–1373.

Department of Health. *Improving Outcomes – A Strategy for Cancer*. Department of Health 2011. http://www.dh.gov.uk/prod_consum_dh/groups/dh_digitalassets/documents/digitalasset/dh_123394.pdf [accessed 10 April 2011].

Hamilton W. Cancer diagnosis in primary care. *Br J Gen Pract* 2010;**60**: 121–128.

Mitchell E, Macdonald S, Cambell N, Weller D, Macleod U. Influences on pre-hospital delay in the diagnosis of colorectal cancer: a systematic review. *Br J Cancer* 2007, 1–11 advance online publication, 4 December 2007; doi:10.1038/sj.bjc.6604096.

NHS Modernisation Agency. Cancer in Primary Care: *A Guide to Good Practice*. 2004. (http://www.cancerimprovement.nhs.uk/documents/good_practice_guide/Good_Practice_Guide.pdf).

NICE *Referral Guidelines for Suspected Cancer in Adults and Children*. Clinical guideline 27. National Institute for Health and Clinical Excellence. www.nice.org.uk June 2005.

CHAPTER 10

Radiotherapy for Rectal Cancer

Andrew Weaver

Department of Oncology, Churchill Hospital, Oxford, UK

OVERVIEW

- Rectal cancer is very common in the UK, with over 13,000 people per year diagnosed
- Radiotherapy treatment may be delivered preoperatively or postoperatively
- When rectal cancer threatens the mesorectal margin, chemoradiotherapy should be administered prior to undertaking surgery
- Preoperative chemoradiotherapy maximises the chance of obtaining complete surgical excision when the mesorectal margin is threatened, maximising local control and the chance of sphincter preservation
- Non-operative therapies are becoming increasingly successful, with increasing response rates prior to surgery

Table 10.1 Rectal cancer symptoms.

Symptoms due to the primary tumour:	Rectal bleeding Change in bowel habit Pelvic pain/obstructive symptoms
Symptoms due to spread of the cancer:	Abdominal/right hypochondrial pain or discomfort Jaundice Cough and shortness of breath
Generalised symptoms of cancer:	Loss of appetite Weight loss Lethargy

of cancer. Patients with rectal cancers may present earlier than patients with colon cancer because the rectal tumours are more often associated with rectal bleeding resulting in patients seeking medical help earlier. Table 10.1.

Diagnosis and staging investigations

The diagnosis is made by taking a full history, clinical examination and investigations including sigmoidoscopy, colonoscopy and biopsy of the tumour for histological confirmation. The tumour is staged by performing an MRI of the pelvis and CT scan of the chest/abdomen and pelvis (see Chapter 8).

MRI scanning is the modality of choice for preoperative staging before surgery or neoadjuvant treatment. If the mesorectal fascia/margin is threatened or invaded by the rectal tumour then the surgeon is unlikely to be able to completely resect the tumour, and consequently risk leaving viable cancer cells behind. If there is more than 2 mm between the advancing tumour edge and the mesorectal margin the surgeon has a high probability of resecting the tumour completely. However, patients with locally advanced tumours (T3/T4) will often require downsizing preoperative chemoradiotherapy. Occasionally involved mesorectal lymph nodes may be situated very close to the mesorectal margin and may compromise the chances of obtaining complete surgical clearance of the tumour without first killing the tumour by preoperative chemoradiotherapy (Figures 10.1 and 10.2).

Introduction

Over 13,000 people in the UK are diagnosed with rectal cancer each year. Three-quarters of these patients will have disease localised to the primary site and for these patients the vast majority will undergo surgery with curative intent. The past decade has seen pronounced changes in the treatment of locally advanced rectal cancer. Historically the standard of care was usually surgery followed by adjuvant radiotherapy or chemoradiotherapy for patients at high risk of relapsing, including those with positive surgical resection margins. More recently patients with locally advanced disease are increasingly being offered neo-adjuvant chemoradiotherapy in order to reduce the size of the cancer (downsize the tumour) thereby making it more likely that the surgeon will be able to completely remove the cancer.

Symptoms

Symptoms may be classified as those caused by the primary tumour, those caused by metastases and those caused by the general effects

Staging of rectal cancer

There are several staging systems in use for colorectal cancer (Table 10.2). These include the Dukes, Astler-Coller, TNM and

---

ABC of Colorectal Cancer, Second Edition.
Edited by Annie Young, Richard Hobbs and David Kerr.
© 2011 Blackwell Publishing Ltd. Published 2011 by Blackwell Publishing Ltd.

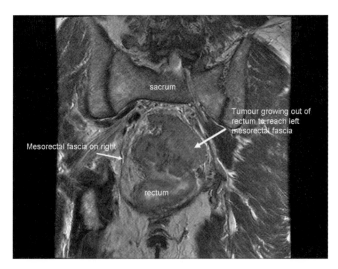

Figure 10.1 Coronal MRI scan of the pelvis showing a huge rectal tumour growing through the rectal wall and threatening the mesorectal margin.

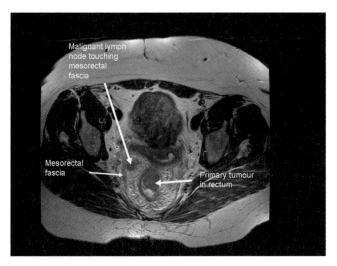

Figure 10.2 Transverse MRI scan of the pelvis showing a rectal tumour and a malignant lymph node next to the rectum that threatens the mesorectal margin.

American Joint Committee on Cancer (AJCC) systems. All these systems describe the spread of the cancer in relation to the layers of the wall of the rectum, organs next to the rectum and organs further away. TNM system describes the extent of the primary **T**umour (T), presence or not of lymph **N**ode metastases (N) and absence or presence of distant **M**etastases (M) (Table 10.2)

Radiotherapy

Radiotherapy has been widely used to prevent local recurrence. The treatment may be given preoperatively or postoperatively. Patients undergoing radiotherapy have a planning CT scan to define the volume of tissue to be irradiated. Generally the clinical target volume encompasses the posterior pelvis to include all identified tumour plus adjacent tissues in the case of preoperative patients, or a similar volume for postoperative patients including the tumour

Table 10.2 Staging for rectal cancer.

	Stage Grouping		
TNM	AJCC	Dukes	Astler-Coller
Tis	0	0	0
T1, T2 N0 M0	Stage I	A	A, B1
T3 N0 M0	Stage IIA	B	B2
T4 N0 M0	Stage IIB	B	B3
T1, T2 N1 M0	Stage IIIA	C	C1
T3, T4 N1 M0	Stage IIIB	C	C2, C3
Any T, N2 M0	Stage IIIC	C	C1, C2, C3
Any T, Any N M1	Stage IV		D

T, primary tumour; Tx, Primary tumour cannot be assessed; T0, No evidence of primary tumour; Tis Carcinoma in situ: intraepithelial or invasion of lamina propria; T1, Tumour invades submucosa; T2, Tumour invades muscularis propria; T3, Tumour invades through muscularis propria into subserosa or into non-peritonealised pericolic or perirectal tissues; T4, Tumour directly invades other organs or structures and/or perforates visceral peritoneum. N, Regional lymph nodes; Nx, Regional lymph nodes cannot be assessed; N0, No regional lymph node metastasis; N1, Metastasis in 1 to 3 regional lymph nodes; N2, Metastasis in 4 or more regional lymph nodes. M, Distant Metastasis; Mx, Distant metastasis cannot be assessed; M0, No distant metastasis; M1, Distant Metastasis.

bed plus adjacent tissues. The inferior border is 3–5 cm below the inferior tumour margin. For mid and upper rectal tumours the anal canal may be spared. The posterior border lies 1 cm behind the anterior border of the sacrum. The anterior border lies 2–3 cm anterior to the sacral promontory. The lateral borders lies 1cm lateral to the pelvic wall. Commonly the defined volume is irradiated by 3 or sometimes 4 fields arranged as a posterior and 2 lateral fields or a posterior, anterior and 2 lateral fields with their central axes crossing at the ioscentre (Figures 10.3 and 10.4). A radiotherapy plan is produced outlining the dose the tumour and normal tissues will receive. To compensate for the curvature of the body, wedge compensators, made of high density metal in the shape

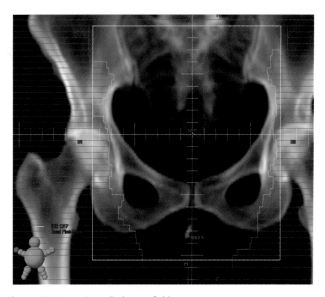

Figure 10.3 Posterior radiotherapy field.

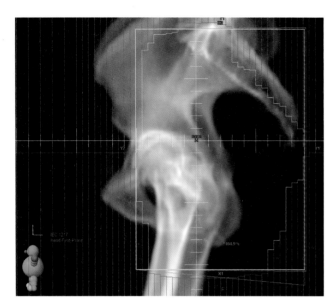

Figure 10.4 Lateral radiotherapy field.

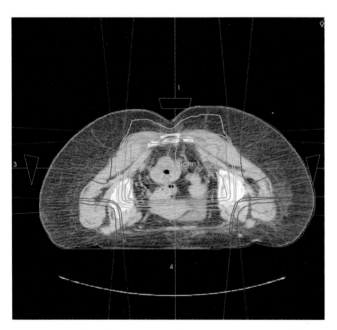

Figure 10.5 Isodose plan.

of a wedge, are inserted into the radiotherapy beam to produce an even dose of radiation across the treatment volume (Figure 10.5).

Standard radiotherapy doses are 45–50 Gy in 25 daily fractions over 5–6 weeks giving between 1.8 Gy and 2 Gy per fraction to the ICRU reference point when combined with chemotherapy.

When patients are unfit for general anaesthesia, or refuse surgery, then higher total tumour doses may need to be considered, ideally attempting to deliver over 70 Gy. However, rectal cancer cannot be treated at this dose with standard external beam radiotherapy and conventional volumes, because rectal and small bowel toxicity would be unacceptable. Endocavitary or interstitial brachytherapy irradiation may be combined with external beam treatment to

achieve doses in excess of 100 Gy. A few groups have demonstrated reasonable results with acceptable acute and long term toxicities using these techniques.

Pre- and postoperative radiotherapy

Despite 15 major prospective randomised trials comparing surgery alone with surgery plus various radiotherapy regimens, the precise role of radiotherapy has yet to be defined. Recent trials using preoperative radiotherapy in patients with rectal cancer have shown significant reductions in local recurrence although only one has shown a clear benefit in terms of improved survival.

The German trial by Saur *et al.* randomised over 823 patients with locally advanced (T3/T4) or node positive rectal cancers to pre- or postoperative chemoradiotherapy. The 5-year local relapse was 6% in the preoperative group versus 13% in the postoperative group (p = 0.006). Both acute (27% vs 40%) and late toxic (14% vs 24%) effects of treatment were significantly increased in those patients receiving postoperative therapy. These results contributed to a paradigm shift, such that preoperative chemoradiotherapy has been widely adopted as the standard of care for locally advanced rectal cancer with postoperative therapy being rarely used in this setting.

Radiotherapy courses given preoperatively may be short course (5 fractions) or long course (20–30 fractions). Short course therapy may be given for mobile operable tumours while long course therapy is required for the more locally advanced and fixed tumours in order to downsize them. The Swedish Rectal Cancer Trial (1997) reported a reduction in overall recurrence at 5 years from 27% following surgery alone to 11% when short course radiotherapy was given prior to surgery. This trial was the first to show an overall improvement in survival (5-year survival 58% for radiotherapy plus surgery compared with 48% for surgery alone [p = 0.004]). Surgery is undertaken within 1 week of completing short course preoperative radiotherapy. While this short course therapy may produce some reduction in tumour bulk, a downstaging effect is not seen. Whether a longer interval between completion of radiotherapy and surgery would lead to a meaningful downsizing effect on the tumour remains unanswered.

Disadvantages of short course preoperative therapy the fact that high radiotherapy doses per fraction (5 Gy per fraction) may result in more severe late (long term) side effects.

Preoperative radiotherapy is not selective and there is little information on which subgroups of patients may benefit e.g. do patients with T1–T2 N0 tumours benefit as much as patients T2–T3 N1 tumours? Table 10.3 outlines some of the early and late side effects which may be experienced by patients undergoing radiotherapy.

Short courses of radiotherapy (up to 10 fractions) may be used to palliate symptoms such as rectal bleeding or bone pain.

Chemotherapy

Recent years have seen key advances regarding the addition of chemotherapy to preoperative radiotherapy. Concomitant chemotherapy with a flouropyrimidine (5-Florouracil or Capecitabine)

Table 10.3 Side effects of radiotherapy.

Early (acute) effects	Late (long term) effects (<5% incidence)
Lethargy	
Skin – erythema, dry, moist desquamation and hair loss	Skin pigmentation or rarely fibrosis, possible permanent hair loss
GI – Diarrhoea and proctitis Abdominal pain	Bowel stricture, perforation, ulceration. Altered bowel habit, incontinence. Pelvic pain
Bladder – Frequency of micturition and dysuria	Incontinence
Early menopause	Infertility, vaginal dryness and vaginal stenosis. Impotence

is the most common approach in order to enhance the local response compared with radiotherapy alone. The combined use of chemoradiotherapy can lead to pathological complete response rates (i.e. no evidence of remaining tumour within the surgically resected specimen) of up to nearly 30% especially if some of the newer chemotherapy agents such as oxaliplatin and irinotecan are added to the chemotherapy regimen. Preoperative trials incorporating new agents such as cetuximab and bevacizumab are currently ongoing.

Future directions

Preoperative chemoradiotherapy for locally advanced rectal tumours has become the standard of care in order to downsize the tumour and make complete surgical excision of the tumour more achievable.

As non-operative treatments for rectal cancer become increasingly successful, overall complete response rates prior to surgery are steadily increasing. It is tempting for those patients achieving a complete response following their chemoradiotherapy to avoid surgery altogether, especially if the surgery involves a permanent colostomy. However, to date, there are no prospective randomised controlled trials to demonstrate this is a safe course of action for patients to follow. Until such evidence becomes available surgery should remain the standard of care for all patients receiving preoperative chemoradiotherapy.

Further reading

The Swedish Rectal Cancer Trial Group, Improved survival with pre-operative radiotherapy in resectable cancer. Swedish Rectal Cancer Trial. *N Engl J Med* 1997;**336**:980–987.

O'Neill BDP, Brown G, Heald RJ, Cunningham D, Tait DM. Non-operative treatment after neoadjuvant chemoradiotherapy for rectal cancer. *Lancet Oncology* 2007;**8**:625–633.

Quirke P, Durdey P, Dixon MF, *et al.* The prediction of local recurrence of rectal adenocarcinoma due to inadequate surgical resection. Histopathological study of lateral tumour spread and surgical excision. *Lancet* 1986;**2**:996–999.

Sauer R, Becker H, Hohenberger W, *et al.* Preoperative versus post operative chemoradiotherapy for rectal cancer. *N Engl J Med* 2004;**351**:1731–1740.

Colorectal Cancer Collaborative Group. Adjuvant radiotherapy for rectal cancer: a systematic overview of 8,507 patients from 22 randomised trials. *Lancet* 2001 Oct 20;**358**(9290):1291–1304.

CHAPTER 11

Surgical Interventions

Shazad Ashraf and Neil Mortensen

Department of Colorectal Surgery, John Radcliffe Hospital, Oxford

---

OVERVIEW

- Current surgical challenges in surgical oncology include the refinement of the techniques that involve the resection of colorectal cancers. The objective is to achieve a negative resection margin as well as minimising the impact on functional outcome and morbidity

- Laparoscopic colorectal surgery is now standard practice at specialist centres with the emergence of novel techniques to reduce the number of incisions and ports

- Although total mesorectal excision is the gold standard for rectal cancers, it is associated with considerable morbidity. Early low-risk rectal cancers may be considered for transanal endoscopic microsurgery, particularly in the elderly

- Metastatic disease is no longer considered a death sentence and improvements in techniques for resection of secondary deposits in the liver and lungs will further increase the group of patients that are suitable for surgery

---

Introduction

Approximately 80% of newly diagnosed cases require surgery, thus accounting for a major component of the workload of colorectal services. As for many cancers, colorectal cancer incidence increases with age, with 83% of cases arising in people over the age of 60 years. This has obvious implications during preoperative evaluation.

Principles of surgery

Box 11.1 summarises the Principles of Colorectal Cancer Surgery. Colorectal cancer is thought to spread in several ways, including direct growth, transperitoneal migration, lymphatic and haematogenous spread and implantation. The aim of surgical resection is to remove all cancerous tissue. Involved margins and lymph nodes are associated with increased risk of recurrence and a worse prognosis. In cases of tumours involving spread to adjacent organs, an en-bloc resection may have to be undertaken to achieve a negative margin.

ABC of Colorectal Cancer, Second Edition.
Edited by Annie Young, Richard Hobbs and David Kerr.
© 2011 Blackwell Publishing Ltd. Published 2011 by Blackwell Publishing Ltd.

Box 11.1 Principles of cancer surgery

Main goals for cancer surgery
- isolation of the tumour
- removal of all tissue containing cancer cells with an adequate margin
- removal of regional lymph nodes
- maintenance of organ function

Additional goals for rectal cancer surgery
- sphincter preservation
- maintenance of sexual function

It is unusual for a tumour to extend distally more than 1 cm from the visible bulk of the tumour. Therefore a minimum distal resection margin of 2 cm is usually sufficient. Radial extension may result in adhesion to adjacent tissues. To achieve mesenteric nodal resection, the arterial trunk is ligated at its origin. Before mobilising the tumour, the lymphovascular bundle is ligated early in order to minimise the release of circulating tumour cells (Figure 11.1).

Rectal cancer surgery is made more difficult due to the pelvic constraints, adjacent genitourinary organs and the presence of the sphincters. The aim is to remove the rectum with its mesorectum and an intact fascial envelope (TME, total mesorectal excision). Breaching this envelope runs the risk of shedding cancer cells into the pelvis (Figure 11.2).

Both sphincter preservation and maintenance of sexual function are of vital importance in rectal cancer surgery. Tumours which are more than 5 cm from the anal verge and do not invade the pelvic floor can be considered for sphincter preserving procedures. However, such surgery comes with significant morbidity and also mortality. Early rectal (T1–T2) tumours (<30 mm) may be suitable for TEM (transanal endoscopic microsurgery), which has much better functional outcomes and is less radical than standard TME (this is discussed later).

Surgical planning

Surgery is considered to be the gold standard in order to achieve complete removal of tumours. Once a cancer is diagnosed, it is important to establish whether it is localised. The presence of distant metastases influences any treatment strategy. Broadly

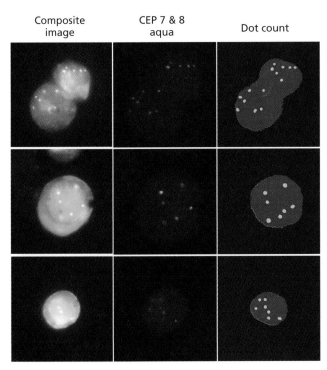

Composite image   CEP 7 & 8 aqua   Dot count

Figure 11.1 Circulating tumour cells isolated from the peripheral blood of a preoperative patient with colorectal cancer. The left of the panel shows the composite images at high magnification (x100) of cells stained with AUA-1 (green fluorescence, EpCAM specific antibody), CAM 5.2 (Cy5 fluorescence, epithelial keratin specific antibody), DAPI (nuclear stain) followed by FISH, with CEP 7/aqua (centromeric probe for chromosome 7) and CEP 8/aqua (centromeric probe for chromosome 8). This demonstrates that these cells are epithelial with a total of 7 aqua dots present in each nucleus, indicating polysomy for at least one of the chromosomes 7 or 8 (the middle panel shows cell images in the aqua channel). A pseudo coloured composite image of the nucleus, in which chromosomes 7 and 8 appear as aqua dots, is shown on the right of the panel (dot count). (Courtesy of Dr. Triantafyllia G. Ntouroupi, Weatherall Institute of Molecular Medicine, Oxford.)

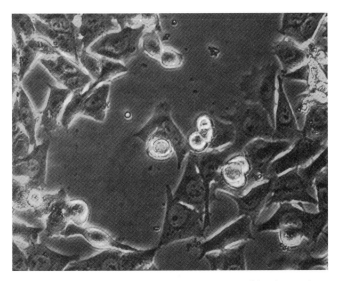

Figure 11.2 A photomicrograph of a colorectal cancer cell line (SKCO-1) established in culture. The line was derived from a human metastatic colorectal cancer. (Courtesy of Sir Walter Bodmer, Weatherall Institute of Molecular Medicine, Oxford.)

speaking, surgery is the first option in colonic lesions. For stage II or III rectal cancer, preoperative radiotherapy with and without chemotherapy is considered prior to resection (Chapter 10). Factors such as the ability of the patient to manage a stoma also need to be considered prior to surgery.

Clinical assessment

It is important to evaluate the stage of the cancer and to exclude synchronous tumours. This will influence whether the tumour is suitable for local or segmental resection. The presence of metastases will influence whether systemic therapy is considered.

Prior to rectal surgery, anorectal function needs to be assessed. In patients with poor function, sphincter preservation will be less of an issue. Past history is also of importance, for example previous radiotherapy for urogenital organs precludes the use of peri-operative radiotherapy. Box 11.2 summarises an example of a medical clinical assessment.

> Box 11.2 **Clinical assessment**
>
> - Establish stage
> - Are there synchronous lesions?
> - Evaluate operative risk
> - Assess preoperative anorectal function
> - Level of tumour from anal verge
> - Imaging (CT/MRI/US)
> - PET scan in cases of recurrence

Preoperative evaluation

Imaging for preoperative staging is detailed in Chapter 8. Routine investigations include the use of blood tests (including FBC, renal function and liver function tests as well as serum CEA) ECG, CXR, chest function and the detection of metastases (CT, CT-PET and MRI).

Assessment of peri-operative risk

A thorough preoperative evaluation in order to minimise the risk of death and morbidity is essential. Patients with chronic diseases such as ischaemic heart disease, congestive cardiac failure, hypertension, asthma and diabetes mellitus need to be optimised prior to surgery. Warfarin, clopidogrel and aspirin need to be stopped and adequate DVT prophylaxis instituted. Transanal excision for rectal cancer is associated with decreased stress on the cardiovascular and respiratory systems and may be a suitable option in patients with significant co-morbidities.

Preoperative preparation

Standard practice is now to omit mechanical bowel preparation. Patients have oral dietary restriction to fluids only and a phosphate enema for rectal and left colonic operations. DVT prophylaxis is important with the use of LMWH and graded compression stockings. Epidural anaesthesia is imperative for postoperative pain control in conventional open surgery. In laparoscopic surgery, a reduction in analgesic requirements has been seen which enables a more rapid recovery programme. Preoperative preparation is outlined in Box 11.3.

Box 11.3 Preoperative preparation

- Preoperative optimisation in patients with chronic diseases (eg heart disease and diabetes)
- Omit warfarin, clopidogrel and aspirin
- DVT prophylaxis
- Dietary restrictions to fluids only
- Phosphate enemas for rectal operations
- Positioning on the operating table
- Rectal washout
- Urinary catheter

Positioning of the patient is dependent on the site of the colorectal lesion. For right and proximal transverse colon tumours, patients are placed in the supine position. Those with left colonic cancers are placed in the Lloyd-Davis position. Rectal irrigation can be carried out in those with rectal tumours. This is done with 0.3% chlorhexidine solution, which has some anti-microbial and tumourcidal properties. A urinary catheter is placed for peri-operative monitoring of kidney function.

Operative access: conventional approach

The incision is placed in order to gain best access to the bowel tumour. A midline incision is most often used. However, transverse incisions, particularly for right colonic cancers, are associated with less pain, improved ventilation of lung bases and better cosmesis postoperatively. Irrespective of the type of incision, a complete laparotomy is performed paying attention to the mobility of the tumour as well as the liver, small bowel, lateral peritoneal spaces and the pelvis.

Table 11.1 describes the types of resections for the tumour location.

Laparoscopic surgery

The first reports of laparoscopic colectomy for cancer were made in the early 1990s. Initial observations of port site metastases were concerning. However, recent meta-analyses (consisting of COST,

Table 11.1 Types of colorectal resections performed.

Operation	Location of tumour
Right hemicolectomy	caecum, right colon, hepatic flexure
Extended right hemicolectomy	transverse colon or splenic flexure
Transverse colectomy	transverse colon
Left hemicolectomy	splenic flexure or left colon
Sigmoid colectomy	sigmoid colon
High anterior resection	rectosigmoid, upper third rectum
Low anterior resection	middle third rectum
Abdominoperineal resection	distal third rectum

MRC-CLASSIC and COLOR trials) have shown that laparoscopic colorectal surgery is as safe and efficacious as the conventional open approach with no difference in overall and disease-free survival. In addition, laparoscopic resection was associated with reductions in peri-operative blood loss, postoperative pain, length of incision and length of hospital stay (2 days) when compared with open surgery. For short-term outcomes, the trials in the meta-analysis found little difference in 30-day mortality and morbidity. The length of time of laparoscopic procedures was found to be longer when compared to the conventional approach. Unsurprisingly, an inverse relationship was found between operating times/complications and the volume of laparoscopic cases carried out at individual centres. For excision of colorectal cancers, laparoscopy should be the preferred method in specialist centres. In centres with considerable laparoscopic expertise, there has been a drive to achieve fewer incisions. This has seen the advent of single-incision laparoscopic surgery (SILS). At present, only around 40% of colorectal surgeons are trained in laparoscopic colorectal surgery, but with the implementation of a national training programme called 'LAPCO', it is expected that this figure will rise over the next 5 years.

Colonic surgery

A right hemicolectomy is the usual operation for right colonic lesions. The colon is mobilised in the avascular plane with preservation of the duodenum, head of the pancreas and the right ureter. In laparoscopy, this is routinely done in a medial-to-lateral approach with early ligation of the ileocolic vessels. The anastomosis can be constructed with hand sutures or staples.

Transverse colonic lesions and splenic flexure carcinoma are managed by an extended right hemicolectomy. For splenic flexure tumours, the left colic artery is ligated at its origin from the inferior mesenteric artery (IMA). The other option is to perform an extended anterior resection with creation of a colorectal anastomosis. Sigmoid cancers can be resected using a left hemicolectomy or sigmoid colectomy. In cases where the tumour has eroded into an adjacent organ, an en-bloc resection is necessary to achieve adequate clearance.

Fifteen per cent of colonic cancers present as surgical emergencies, with either obstruction or perforation. In the emergency setting, complications are substantial and are probably secondary to disturbances in fluid balance and the presence of septic complications. The overall mortality for an obstructing cancer is around 20%. Left colonic tumours are usually managed with a resection and formation of colostomy. In some instances, obstructing sigmoid and left colonic tumours can be managed in the acute situation by endoscopic insertion of colonic stents. This provides a temporising measure prior to definitive surgery, which can be done after an interval of a few weeks, allowing for improvement in patient condition.

Rectal surgery

Mobilisation of rectum

Immediately before resection, a EUA (examination under anaesthesia) is carried out to locate the tumour and confirm the exact type of operation to be performed. The patient is positioned in the Lloyd-Davis position. The left colon and mesentery are dissected off the retroperitoneum and the left ureter identified. The IMA is doubly ligated and divided with preservation of the autonomic nerves (responsible for ejaculation and erection). In laparoscopy, a medial-to-lateral approach is employed with early isolation of the IMA bundle. TME involves removing the rectum together with an intact mesorectum. Utilisation of this technique has been associated with lower recurrence rates.

The mobilised rectum is then divided after application of a transverse stapling device and proximal bowel clamp below the tumour. A circular stapling device is then placed in the rectal stump to fashion an end-to-end anastomosis. Its integrity can be checked by the retrieval of complete donuts and a negative leak test. If the level of the anastomosis is low, then a defunctioning stoma is fashioned, which can then be subsequently closed after 3 months.

Abdominoperineal resection

This involves the removal of low rectal cancers together with the sphincter complex; usually for tumours less than 5 cm from the anal verge. The anal canal, rectum and the distal sigmoid colon are removed. The abdominal part of the operation can be done laparoscopically. The operation is then completed via a perineal incision. The specimen can be removed through this incision, thus avoiding the need for an abdominal incision. An end colostomy is fashioned in the left iliac fossa. Perineal wound dehiscence can be particularly troublesome postoperatively, particularly after neoadjuvant radiotherapy.

Local treatment of colorectal cancer

Adenomatous polyps and early rectal tumours may be suitable for local resection. Transanal endoscopic microsurgery (TEM) uses a closed operating proctoscope to visualise the rectum. The rectum is insufflated with CO_2 and the polyp is excised using a full thickness or partial thickness approach. If there is a suspicion of cancer, a full wall thickness incision can be employed. The wall can be left open if the defect is low and posterior in the rectum due to its relation to the peritoneum. Transanal excision in the submucosal plane can be used for large circumferential rectal lesions that are less than 10 cm from the dentate line.

TEM is far superior to radical surgery (TME) with regards to functional outcomes. These include urinary incontinence, sexual dysfunction and bowel frequency/incontinence. Most patients are discharged within 24–48 hours following TEM. The complication rate is far lower for TEM when compared to TME. A key factor in determining the success of TEM in early rectal cancer is the knowledge of lymph node metastasis. In this regard, TEM has a limited capacity to remove lymph nodes in the mesorectum, unlike TME. T1 cancers have been reported to have a metastasis rate between 0 and 15%. Current imaging modalities are not sensitive enough to detect such lesions preoperatively with a high level of

certainty. Follow-up is extremely important in detecting local or systemic recurrence, as control can be achieved by salvage radical resection (Chapter 16). Interestingly, a prospective, randomised study (n = 52) showed no significant difference in 5-year survival, local recurrence rate and metastasis rate between patients with T1 tumours that had been treated by TEM or TME. A recent randomised trial (TREC) has been set up to compare outcomes for those undergoing short-course radiotherapy and TEM versus radical surgery in early rectal cancers (T1–T2).

Metastatic surgery

The published literature on outcomes for resections of colorectal liver metastases demonstrates reasonable 5-year survivals (25–44%) and operative mortality, which range from (0–6%). The main complications from this type of surgery are liver failure (secondary to the extent of resection or presence of underlying liver disease), haemorrhage, biliary leaks, sepsis and cardiopulmonary problems. As for any oncological surgery, resection margins are important, with some evidence from the Registry of Hepatic Metastases that shows that a margin less than 1 cm is associated with poor outcome. Lesions that are not resectable can undergo cryotherapy or radiofrequency ablation. Solitary pulmonary lesions can also be resected with comparatively good outcomes.

Conclusion

Surgery remains the mainstay of treatment for patients with colorectal cancer in addition to neoadjuvant and adjuvant therapy. Laparoscopic colorectal surgery is now an established technique and is performed routinely in specialist centres with good outcomes. Experienced laparoscopic surgeons are even endeavouring to carry out resections through single small incisions. Although TME is the gold standard, TEM should be considered a treatment option for early rectal cancers. Future studies will further evaluate both cancer-related and functional outcomes for these two techniques.

Further reading

Bai H, Chen B, Zhou Y and Wu X, Five-year long-term outcomes of laparoscopic surgery for colon cancer. *World J Gastroenterol* 2010 October 21;**16**(39):4992–4997.

Garden OJ, *et al.*, Guidelines for resection of colorectal cancer liver metastases. *Gut*, 2006;**55** Suppl 3: p. iii1–8.

Heald RJ, Husband EM, and Ryall RD, The mesorectum in rectal cancer surgery–the clue to pelvic recurrence ? *Br J Surg*, 1982;**69**(10): 613–616.

Ho YH and Ooi LL, Recent advances in the total management of colorectal cancer. *Ann Acad Med Singapore*, 2003;**32**(2):143–144.

Motson RW, Laparoscopic surgery for colorectal cancer. *Br J Surg*, 2005;**92**(5): 519–520.

Scholefield JH and Steele RJ, Guidelines for follow up after resection of colorectal cancer. *Gut*, 2002. **51** Suppl 5:V3–5.

Turnbull RB, *et al.*, Cancer of the colon: the influence of the no-touch isolation technic on survival rates. *CA Cancer J Clin*, 1968;**18**(2):82–87.

CHAPTER 12

Adjuvant Therapy

Zenia Saridaki-Zoras[1] *and David Kerr*[2]

[1]Laboratory of Tumor Cell Biology, Medical School, University of Crete, Crete, Greece
[2]University of Oxford, Oxford, UK

OVERVIEW

- The role of adjuvant therapy is to reduce any residual micrometastatic disease left in the body after surgery in an attempt to improve the cure rates
- Oxaliplatin-based chemotherapy (preferably with infusional 5-FU/LV) for 6 months initiated within 8 weeks after surgery is the standard of care for stage III colon cancer
- Oral fluoropyrimidines have shown equivalent efficacy and safety to IV infusion of 5-FU/LV
- Monoclonal antibodies (such as bevacizumab and cetuximab) have failed in the adjuvant setting, as has the chemotherapy, irinotecan
- Adjuvant therapy for stage II colon cancer remains controversial, defective DNA Mismatch Repair (dMMR) could be used for selection of patients with an excellent prognosis that will not benefit in absolute terms from adjuvant 5FU/LV chemotherapy, but 5-FU/LV can be offered to patients with good performance status or markers associated with a higher risk of recurrence

Introduction

Of the global burden of 1 million new colorectal cancer cases each year, approximately 400,000 patients die in the same period of time. Despite the clear progress made in surgical techniques, the risk of recurrence for the 70–80% of the newly diagnosed patients who present with localised disease is still high. Recurrence, after potentially curative resection with no evidence of macroscopic residual tumour, is thought to originate from clinically and radiologically occult microscopic dissemination present before surgery. Adjuvant treatment in the form of chemotherapy has become the main tool to target and eradicate micrometastatic disease. Substantial progress has been made in this field over the last few decades, and a number of new drugs, such as oxaliplatin and oral fluoropyrimidines, have been added to the traditional chemotherapeutic armamentarium, 5-fluorouracil (5-FU) and leucovorin (LV).

ABC of Colorectal Cancer, Second Edition.
Edited by Annie Young, Richard Hobbs and David Kerr.
© 2011 Blackwell Publishing Ltd. Published 2011 by Blackwell Publishing Ltd.

Which endpoints define clinical benefit?

It has been shown that in stage III colon cancer, adjuvant chemotherapy has produced a statistically significant and clinically meaningful reduction in recurrence rate and improvement in overall survival (OS) compared to surgery alone. OS, usually reported 5 years from the tumour resection, has traditionally been the gold standard assessment of adjuvant treatment. However, as a primary endpoint, it needs long follow-up, may delay the incorporation of novel effective agents in the adjuvant setting and could be influenced by subsequent salvage therapy for recurrent disease, potentially obscuring the value of any new, adjuvant intervention. Recently, 3-year disease-free survival (DFS) has been shown to correlate highly with 5-year OS and, consequently, it can be used as a 'clean' surrogate endpoint to define relative benefit from any new adjuvant treatment.

Conventional therapy with leucovorin-modulated 5-FU

For nearly 50 years now fluoropyrimidines, and in particular intravenous (IV) 5-FU, have been the mainstay of chemotherapy for a large spectrum of solid tumours, including colorectal cancer.

The optimal dose of LV and the levamisole contribution was addressed in the 'certain arm' of QUASAR (Quick And Simple And Reliable) trial. The results showed that neither levamisole, nor high dose LV, contributed to improved survival. At least three randomised trials have shown no additional benefit from 12 instead of 6 months of 5-FU/LV, thus, with improved DFS at 3 years and a 5–6% absolute improvement in 5 year survival, the combination of 5-FU/LV for 6 months had become standard of care in adjuvant stage III colon cancer patients.

There are some clinical data for advanced CRC to suggest that prolonged 5-FU/LV infusion has an improved safety and efficacy profile compared with the bolus delivery (e.g. 'Roswell Park' and 'Mayo Clinic' regimens). However, in the adjuvant setting, randomised clinical trials showed no statistically significant differences in DFS and OS, but the toxicity profile was more favourable for continuous infusion, with significantly less severe diarrhoea, mucositis and neutropenia. This toxicity profile may be offset by the inconvenience associated with central venous lines, pumps and additional treatment delivery costs.

Oral fluoropyrimidines

Capecitabine is an oral fluoropyrimidine designed to generate 5-FU preferentially at the tumour bed, as is UFT, a 4:1 molar combination of ftorafur with uracil which achieves higher 5-FU concentrations in both tumour and plasma.

The X-ACT trial randomly assigned 1987 stage III colon cancer patients after surgery to 6 months of capecitabine monotherapy or bolus 5-FU/LV (Mayo regimen). There was some suggestion of superiority of the capecitabine arm with a 3-year DFS – Table 12.1. Adjuvant UFT versus bolus IV 5-FU/LV (Roswell Park schedule) was compared in the NSABP C-06 trial. No difference was shown in 5-year DFS and 5-year OS between the two arms – Table 12.1. These studies have established the place of oral fluoropyrimidines as a basis of new adjuvant regimens that seem to be more convenient to patients with an overall favourable toxicity profile.

Combination chemotherapy

The MOSAIC study was the first to suggest a benefit from the addition of oxaliplatin to 5-FU adjuvant chemotherapy: 2,246 stage II and stage III colon cancer patients were randomly assigned to receive either FOLFOX4 or infusional 5-FU and leucovorin (de Gramont regimen) – Figure 12.1. The 3-year DFS, the trial's primary endpoint, was significantly higher with FOLFOX4 – Table 12.2. In a subgroup analysis, the DFS benefit reached the level of statistical significance among stage III but not stage II patients. After 6 years of follow-up, OS benefit is limited to stage III patients – Table 12.2. Despite oxaliplatin showing improved efficacy compared to 5-FU/LV, this comes at a price of increased toxicity. Peripheral neuropathy was present in 92% of patients

Table 12.1 Oral fluoropyrimidines in the adjuvant treatment setting of colon cancer patients.

Trial	Stage	No. of patients	DFS	OS
X-ACT (FU/LV vs capecitabine)	III	1987	**3y** 60.6% vs 64.2% (p 0.05)	**3y** 77.6% vs 81.3% (p 0.07)
NSABP C-06 (FU/LV vs UFT/LV)	II/III	1608	**5y** 66.9% vs 68.3% (p 0.79)	**5y** 78.7% vs 78.7% (p 0.88)

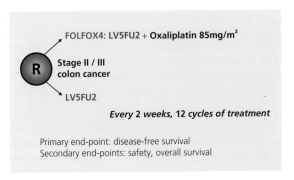

Figure 12.1 MOSAIC study design.

Table 12.2 Oxaliplatin combination chemotherapy in the adjuvant treatment of patients with colon cancer.

Trial	Stage	No. of patients	DFS	OS
MOSAIC (inf FU/LV vs FOLFOX4)	II/III	2246	**3y** 69.8% vs 76.4% (p < 0.001)	**4y** 82.8% vs 84.9%
			5y 67.4% vs 73.5% (p 0.003)	**6y** 75.8% vs 78.5%
NSABP C-07 (bolus FU/LV vs FLOX)	II/III	2492	**3y** 71.6% vs 76.5% (p 0.004)	

during treatment but it was generally reversible. Improved DFS was also reported in the NSABP C-07 trial with the addition of oxaliplatin to bolus 5-FU/LV, but toxicity was prominent in both groups – Table 12.2. Furthermore, in the NO16968/XELOXA study in which stage III CRC patients were randomised to receive either oral capecitabine plus oxaliplatin or fluorouracil and folinic acid, a 3-year DFS improvement with the triple combination (70.9% vs 66.5%, HR 0.80) but a non-significant 5-year benefit in OS (3.4%) were documented. Based on these results, oxaliplatin-containing regimens should be considered for stage III colon cancer patients who can tolerate the potential long term peripheral neuropathy. Bearing in mind toxicity considerations as well, fluoropyrimidine monotherapy should be considered as the treatment of choice for the elderly stage III CRC patients.

In contrast to its use in advanced disease, no significant improvement in DFS and OS has been shown with adjuvant irinotecan added to fluorouracil in 3 randomised trials. Therefore, at present, the use of irinotecan in the management of early disease is not justified.

The International Duration Evaluation of Adjuvant chemotherapy (IDEA) trial and the SCOT study in the UK is currently recruiting patients to investigate the optimal duration of combination chemotherapy (3 vs 6 months) in the adjuvant setting; something that, if proven, could be of striking importance for patients and healthcare providers.

Stage II colon cancer

In contrast to the clear overall survival benefit of 8–10% given by adjuvant chemotherapy to patients with stage III disease, its role in stage II is still controversial and no international consensus has been reached regarding its use. Approximately 80% of stage II colon cancer patients will be cured by surgery alone and the lack of large and adequately powered clinical trials in stage II disease has led to data collection from prospectively defined subgroups of existing trials. Such trials, in which a mixture of stage II and III patients were included, failed to demonstrate a significant survival benefit from 5-FU adjuvant chemotherapy in stage II patients. Meta-analysis and pooled analysis also failed to show any survival advantage. The ASCO guidelines recommend against routine administration of 5-FU based chemotherapy for medically fit stage II patients. Nevertheless, it is suggested that several subsets of patients defined as high risk can be excluded – Box 12.1. The recently revised American Joint Committee of Cancer further stratifies stage II and III disease using data from SEER (Surveillance, Epidemiology and End Results) and demonstrate that 5-year survival was statistically significantly better for stage IIIa than for stage IIb (T4) patients – Figure 12.4.

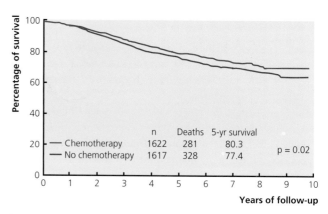

Figure 12.3 QUASAR study. OS in the intention to treat population (ITT).

> **Box 12.1 ASCO recommendations for stage II colon cancer patients**
>
> Patients with:
>
> - poorly differentiated histology
> - T4 lesions
> - bowel perforation at presentation
> - inadequately sampled lymph nodes (n < 13)
>
> are considered high risk and if medically fit can be offered 5-FU based adjuvant chemotherapy
>
> - Very important: patient's choice in the treatment decision-making process after information regarding risk of recurrence/death and possible side effects from chemotherapy are supplied by the oncologist

The largest randomised trial (n = 3200) of stage II adjuvant chemotherapy is the QUASAR 'uncertain' study – Figure 12.2. With a median follow-up of 4.6 years, adjuvant chemotherapy was associated with significantly reduced recurrence – Figure 12.3. The 5 year survival benefit of 3–4% for chemotherapy was also significant (p = 0.04) among stage II colon cancer patients. These new data suggest that it is reasonable to discuss the small benefits associated with chemotherapy with individual patients to make an informed decision about their own treatment.

Selecting those patients that would benefit based on predictive molecular factors (like TS expression, 18q deletion, p53 mutation, gene expression profile) is an area of active ongoing research as covered in Chapter 3. Patient characterisation of MMR status could provide a more tailored approach towards personalised adjuvant

therapy, and, especially in stage II CRC patients, it could be used to decide who should be considered for adjuvant fluorouracil treatment.

Adjuvant therapy for rectal cancer

The use of adjuvant chemotherapy for rectal cancer is still contentious. No survival benefit was shown with postoperative fluorouracil-based chemotherapy in the EORTC 22921 trial. Nevertheless, in a subsequent unplanned post hoc analysis, it was shown that odd prognosis patients (categorised as ypT0-2) after preoperative chemoradiation had a significant improvement in DFS and OS. In addition, in the QUASAR trial, where approximately 30% of the patients had rectal cancer (948 patients in total), both DFS and OS were statistically significantly greater with the administration of adjuvant chemotherapy. From extrapolation of data from the colon cancer trials, adjuvant chemotherapy is usually administered in rectal cancer patients, although patients exhibit impaired tolerability when preoperative chemoradiation has preceded the chemotherapy alone.

'Adjuvant' chemotherapy after resection of liver metastases

Approximately 30% of patients who have undergone surgical resection for hepatic metastases remain alive 5 years later and two thirds of them are disease free. Although there is a clear survival benefit from resection for carefully selected patients with limited metastatic disease in very few randomised trials, the possible benefit of systemic 5-FU based chemotherapy after hepatic resection has been addressed directly and a clear survival benefit has not yet emerged. Trials with IV regimens containing newer agents, such as oxaliplatin and irinotecan, are much needed. Furthermore, in the EORTC Intergroup trial 40983 where the issue of peri-operative chemotherapy with FOLFOX4 was addressed, it was shown that patients who finally underwent liver resection had an absolute increase in progression-free survival rate at 3 years of 9.2% (HR 0.71, p = 0.025). Cetuximab (see next section) given with 5-fluorouracil, folinic acid and oxaliplatin is recommended as a possible first line treatment for people with metastatic colorectal cancer in the UK,

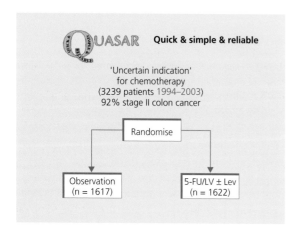

Figure 12.2 QUASAR: Quick and simple and reliable.

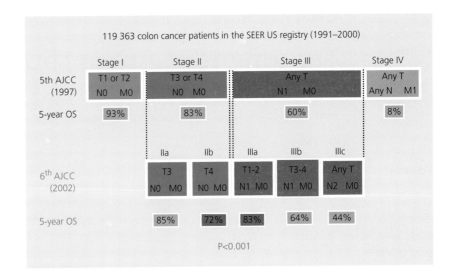

Figure 12.4 Five-year colon cancer survival by stages according to the 6th AJCC edition system with data from the SEER (Surveillance, Epidemiology and End Results) registry (1991–2000).

only when surgery to remove the cancer in the colon or rectum has been carried out or is possible *and the metastases are only in the liver* and cannot be removed surgically before treatment.

Regional therapy, in the form of hepatic intra-arterial chemotherapy (HIA) of fluoropyrimidines, as an adjuvant strategy, has been evaluated in a number of trials. HIA with systemic chemotherapy was evaluated in a number of studies, mostly conducted in the USA. HIA floxuridine (FUDR) plus systemic 5-FU/LV was initially associated with significantly better 2-year liver free disease recurrence (90% vs 60%) and 2-year survival rate (86% vs 72%), but a later report suggested that this benefit may be limited to the high risk subgroup of patients. Recent studies are evaluating HIA with capecitabine, oxaliplatin and irinotecan containing regimens. But, HIA has increased morbidity, is complex and costly, may complicate standard hepatectomy and the initially encouraging results may not be highly reproducible in non-specialised centres.

Future directions and challenges in adjuvant chemotherapy

Monoclonal antibodies have already shown efficacy in metastatic disease, such as cetuximab and bevacizumab – see Chapter 14. However, the adjuvant mFOLFOX6 ± cetuximab N0147 study in stage III CRC patients showed no improvement in DFS and OS for the chemotherapy-antibody arm combination, whereas toxicity was greater in this arm. Furthermore, the 3-year DFS in the adjuvant mFOLFOX6 ± bevacizumab NSABP C-08 study in stage II-III CRC patients was not statistically significantly different between the two arms, but grade 3 adverse events were greater with bevacizumab. The AVANT study – chemotherapy +/− bevacizumab in the adjuvant treatment of early-stage colon cancer, did not meet its primary endpoint of improving disease-free survival in stage III colon cancer; preliminary efficacy data from AVANT numerically favour chemotherapy alone (the control arm).

Many challenges and questions remain to be answered in the adjuvant treatment setting, such as the integration of molecular markers in the prognostic classification and in the identification of high risk stage II patients suitable for treatment and the evaluation

of shorter treatment duration (3 months vs 6 months) in order to minimize oxaliplatin toxicity – Box 12.2. There are now global, cooperative trial networks which work together so that large numbers of patients can be recruited rapidly to define the role of these new approaches.

Box 12.2 **Challenges in the adjuvant treatment setting**

- Identification of high risk stage II patients (molecular markers, gene expression profiles – microarrays and/or Q-RT-PCR)
- Incorporation of molecular targeted therapies based on strong preclinical and clinical rational for high risk patient
- Adjuvant treatment cannot salvage patients from inadequate surgery
- Identification of genetic determinants of toxicity and efficacy (single nucleotide polymorphisms)
- Can the length of adjuvant chemotherapy be further reduced?

Further reading

Andre T, Boni C, Mounedji-Boudiaf L, *et al.* Oxaliplatin, fluorouracil, and leucovorin as adjuvant treatment for colon cancer. *N Engl J Med* 2004;**350**: 2343–2351.

Clark J. Adjuvant therapy for resected colon cancer. UpToDate 15.1 online (©2010 UpToDate® www.uptodate.com).

Chau I and Cunningham D. Adjuvant therapy in colon cancer – what, when and how ? *Annals of Oncology* 2006;**17**:1347–1359.

Gray RG, Kerr DJ, McConkey CC, *et al.* On behalf of QUASAR Collaborative Group. Comparison of fluorouracil with additional levamisole, higher-dose folinic acid, or both, as adjuvant chemotherapy for colorectal cancer: a randomised trial. *The Lancet* 2000;**355**:1588–1596.

Gray, RG, Barnwell J, McConkey C, Williams N, Kerr, DJ. QUASAR: a randomised study of adjuvant chemotherapy versus observation including 3239 colorectal cancer patients QUASAR Collaborative Group. *The Lancet* in Press.

Van Cutsem E, Tejpar S, Verslype C, Laurent S. Challenges in the adjuvant treatment for patients with stages II and III colon cancer. In: *ASCO Educational Book* 2006.

CHAPTER 13

Treatment of Advanced Disease

David Watkins and David Cunningham

Royal Marsden Hospital, London and Surrey, UK

OVERVIEW

- The term 'advanced disease' is used to describe a broad group of patients presenting with either locally advanced or metastatic colorectal cancer
- The availability of combination chemotherapy regimens has had a significant impact on the outcomes of patients with advanced disease
- The majority of patients receive treatment with palliative intent. In selected cases a curative approach using multi-modality therapy may be feasible
- Molecular targeted chemotherapy agents and predictive biomarkers will play an increasing role in the future care of patients with advanced colorectal cancer

---

Table 13.1 Presenting symptoms.

Primary tumour	Change in bowel habit
	Abdominal pain
	Rectal bleeding
	Symptoms of bowel obstruction
Metastatic disease	Liver capsule pain arising from liver deposits
	Cough, breathlessness from lung metastases
	Bloating, obstruction from peritoneal disease
	Abdominal swelling from ascites
General symptoms	Fatigue
	Anorexia
	Weight loss

Introduction

Advanced colorectal cancer represents a significant global disease burden. Of patients diagnosed with colorectal cancer, 20–25% are found to have advanced disease at the time of initial presentation. In addition, a proportion of patients who undergo curative resection of their primary tumour will subsequently develop recurrent disease. The 5-year survival rate for patients with advanced colorectal cancer is approximately 10%. During the past 10 years the treatment paradigms for patients with advanced colorectal cancer have undergone considerable development. The increased availability of active chemotherapy drugs, improved access to specialist care and advances in imaging and surgical techniques have all contributed to improving patient outcomes.

The term 'advanced colorectal cancer' is applied to patients with inoperable primary disease without distant spread (locally advanced) and also to patients with distant sites of disease involvement (metastatic disease). Patients commonly present with symptoms arising from the primary tumour, with the diagnosis of advanced disease only being made on subsequent imaging investigations. A small proportion of patients present with symptoms relating to the presence of metastatic disease (Table 13.1). All

patients diagnosed with colorectal cancer undergo CT imaging of the thorax, abdomen and pelvis to define the extent of disease. In selected cases, particularly where a curative treatment strategy is being considered, MRI or PET imaging may be used to provide further information as to the sites and extent of disease involvement. The commonest site of distant spread is the liver, which is involved in more than 70% of patients with metastatic disease. In approximately 25% of patients the liver is found to be the only site of metastatic spread. Other common sites of involvement include the lungs, peritoneum and lymph nodes. Metastatic spread to bone or the central nervous system is infrequent.

Treatment strategies and the MDT process

In the UK, patients with advanced colorectal cancer are treated in specialist units by multidisciplinary teams (Chapter 6). For the majority of patients with advanced disease treatment is palliative in nature, aimed at improving disease related symptoms and prolonging survival. In a proportion of patients, most notably those with limited metastatic involvement of the liver, lungs or locally advanced rectal tumours, a curative treatment strategy utilising multi-modality therapy may be adopted. Multidisciplinary team meetings play an important role in defining the optimal treatment strategy for individual patients. In selected cases input from hepatic surgeons, interventional radiologists or thoracic surgeons may be required (Table 13.2). Factors taken into consideration when formulating a treatment strategy include: sites of disease involvement, extent of disease, symptomatology, general physical

ABC of Colorectal Cancer, Second Edition.
Edited by Annie Young, Richard Hobbs and David Kerr.
© 2011 Blackwell Publishing Ltd. Published 2011 by Blackwell Publishing Ltd.

Table 13.2 The multidisciplinary team.

Core team	Radiologist with GI radiology expertise
	Histopathologist
	Medical Oncologist
	Clinical Oncologist
	Colorectal Surgeon
	Palliative Care Specialist
	Clinical Nurse Specialist
	Research Nurse
Extended team	Liver Surgeon
	Thoracic Surgeon
	Gastroenterologist
	Interventional Radiologist

Table 13.3 The Eastern Cooperative Oncology Group (ECOG) performance status.

ECOG score	Clinical status
0	Fully active, able to carry out all pre-disease activities without restriction
1	Restricted in physically strenuous activity but ambulatory and able to carry out work of a light or sedentary nature, e.g. light house work, office work
2	Ambulatory and capable of all self-care but unable to carry out any work activities. Up and about more than 50% of waking hours
3	Capable of only limited self-care, confined to bed or chair more than 50% of waking hours
4	Completely disabled. Cannot carry out any self-care. Totally confined to bed or chair

condition (measured by performance status, see Table 13.3), age and co-morbidites.

Treatment strategies for locally advanced disease

Locally advanced disease is frequently encountered in patients with rectal tumours due to the close proximity of the surrounding pelvic structures. In approximately 25% of cases clear resection margins are not attainable with surgery alone and preoperative chemoradiotherapy (radiotherapy with concomitant chemotherapy) is considered.

The use of staging pelvic MRI allows the identification of patients at risk of circumferential resection margin involvement who benefit from preoperative therapy. Chemoradiotherapy can induce tumour regression and allow for clear resection margins to be achieved in many patients initially considered unsuitable for surgical resection (Figure 13.1). Chemotherapy and radiotherapy also play an important palliative role in patients where curative surgery is not feasible. Locally advanced disease involving the colon may infiltrate other intra-abdominal viscera such as the small bowel or spleen, in some cases en bloc resection of the tumour and attached viscera may be undertaken. The use of chemotherapy to attempt to reduce disease bulk prior to attempt at resection may also be considered.

Potentially resectable metastatic disease

Approximately 10–15% of patients with metastatic colorectal cancer have disease that is limited to a small number of deposits (1–4) within a single organ, most commonly the liver or lungs. In this patient population the surgical resection of metastatic deposits can potentially result in cure, with reported 5-year survival rates of 20–40%.

A further group of patients present with metastatic disease that is confined to the liver but is initially considered too extensive for resection. Studies have demonstrated that in a proportion of cases the use of combination chemotherapy can reduce the disease bulk allowing for resection to be undertaken. For appropriately selected patients, long-term survival may approach that of patients with initially resectable liver disease (Figure 13.2).

Chemotherapy for advanced disease

A variety of chemotherapeutic options are now available for use in the management of patients with advanced colorectal cancer. These include both conventional cytotoxic agents and the more recently introduced novel molecular targeted therapies.

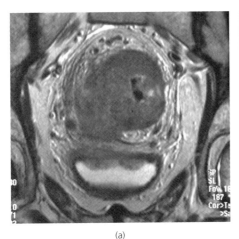
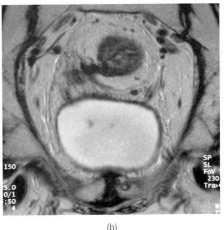

(a)   (b)

Figure 13.1 MRI of a patient with locally advanced rectal cancer. Following preoperative chemoradiotherapy a partial response was achieved allowing for surgical resection to be undertaken. a) Pre treatment MRI; b) Post chemoradiotherapy MRI.

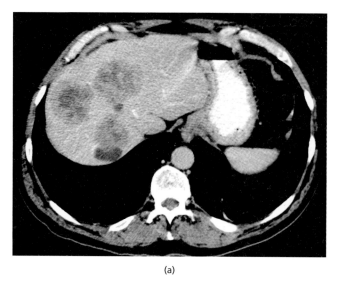

(a)

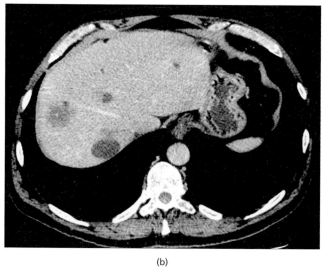

(b)

Figure 13.2 Metastatic disease isolated to the liver. CT image of a patient presenting with large metastatic deposits within the liver and no other sites of disease. A partial response is achieved following 4 cycles of combination chemotherapy allowing for liver resection to be undertaken. Portal vein embolisation has been used to increase the remnant liver volume.

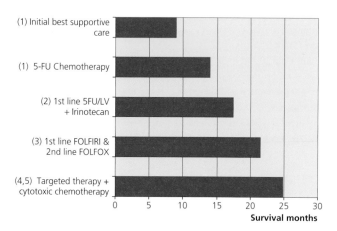

Figure 13.3 Incremental gains in survival have been achieved through the development of combination chemotherapy regimens, second-line therapies and the introduction of molecular targeted agents. The median survival achieved in pivotal first-line studies is shown. See Table 13.5 for references 1–5.

The availability of cytotoxic combination therapies utilising 5-Fluorouracil (5-FU) with either oxaliplatin or irinotecan has been a significant factor contributing to improved patient survival (Figure 13.3). A number of treatment schedules are in regular use, each with differing side effect profiles and levels of anti-tumour activity (Table 13.4). Chemotherapy is most commonly delivered with palliative intent, aiming to provide symptomatic benefit, prolong survival and improve quality of life. Combination chemotherapy schedules are reasonably tolerated and commonly delivered in the palliative setting. In selected cases where the disease is not amenable to metastectomy, single agent first-line therapy with an oral fluoropyrimidine such as capecitabine may be used, particularly in patients with small volume slowly progressive disease, asymptomatic disease or where there is concern about

potential chemotherapy toxicities. Chemotherapy treatment is not routinely recommended for patients with incapacitating disease related fatigue (performance status 3 or 4), where treatment related toxicities may further exacerbate their condition.

Many treatment related side effects can be controlled through the use of supportive therapies and dose reductions where necessary. Patients may present to their GP and it is important that primary care teams are made aware of potential treatment related toxicities patients may experience. A majority of chemotherapy drugs are thrombogenic and many can affect fertility, which may be relevant in some patients.

Treatment response is formally assessed by repeat CT imaging, usually undertaken after 2–3 months of therapy. Changes in symptoms and serum tumour markers may also provide an indication of treatment response. In the palliative setting chemotherapy treatment may be continued providing that side effects remain tolerable and disease progression is not seen. For patients who respond, a treatment break is often considered following completion of 6 months of treatment. Patients with disease progression during initial chemotherapy will be considered for further treatment with alternative regimens (second-line chemotherapy).

5-Fluorouracil (5-FU)

5-FU is a pyrimidine analogue which acts through the inhibition of the enzyme thymidylate synthase. Intravenous 5-FU is administered by either bolus injection or by infusion. Intravenous leucovorin (LV) is often given with intravenous 5-FU to enhance activity. Orally administered 5-FU prodrugs, such as capecitabine, are available which obviate the need for regimens given by prolonged intravenous infusion. Common toxicities include; diarrhoea, palmar plantar erythema and stomatitis. Coronary artery spasm may occur in 2–5% of cases and presents with anginal chest pain. Hair loss is unusual (Figure 13.4 PPE)

Table 13.4 Common chemotherapy schedules.

Chemotherapy	Clinical Setting	Administration
Capecitabine	First line	Tablets taken orally days 1–14 every 21 days
Oxaliplatin + Capecitabine	First or subsequent line	Oxaliplatin as a 2-hour infusion on day 1 with oral capecitabine taken on days 1–14. Repeated every 3 weeks
Oxaliplatin + 5-FU/LV (FOLFOX)	First or subsequent line	Oxaliplatin + LV as a 2-hour infusion followed by 5-FU bolus and 46-hour 5-FU infusion. Repeated every 2 weeks
Irinotecan + 5-FU/LV (FOLFIRI)	First or subsequent line	Irinotecan + LV as a 2-hour infusion followed by 5-FU bolus and 46-hour 5-FU infusion. Repeated every 2 weeks
Irinotecan	Second or subsequent line	Intravenous infusion given every 3 weeks
Bevacizumab	First or subsequent line	Intravenous infusion given every 2 or 3 weeks. Given in conjunction with cytotoxic chemotherapy
Cetuximab	First or subsequent line	Intravenous infusion given every week either as a single agent (3rd line) or in conjunction with cytotoxic chemotheraphy (1st, 2nd and 3rd line)

Table 13.5 Pivotal clinical studies in advanced colorectal cancer.

(1) Nordic Gastrointestinal Tumor Adjuvant Therapy Group. Expectancy or primary chemotherapy in patients with advanced asymptomatic colorectal cancer: a randomized trial. *J Clin Oncol* 1992;**10**(6):904–911.

(2) Douillard J, Cunningham D, Roth A *et al.* Irinotecan combined with fluorouracil compared with fluorouracil alone as first-line treatment for metastatic colorectal cancer: a multicentre randomised trial. *The Lancet* 2000;**355**(9209):1041–1047.

(3) Tournigand C, Andre T, Achille E, Lledo G *et al.* FOLFIRI followed by FOLFOX6 or the reverse sequence in advanced colorectal cancer: a randomized GERCOR study. *J Clin Oncol* 2004;**22**(2):229–37.
  ○ Cunningham D, Humblet Y, Siena S *et al.* Cetuximab monotherapy and cetuximab plus irinotecan in irinotecan-refractory metastatic colorectal cancer. *N Engl J Med* 2004;**351**(4):337-45.
  ○ Hurwitz H, Fehrenbacher L, Novotny W *et al.* Bevacizumab plus irinotecan, fluorouracil, and leucovorin for metastatic colorectal cancer. *N Engl J Med* 2004;**350**(23):2335–2342.

(4) Van Cutsem E, Köhne CH, Hitre E *et al.* Cetuximab and chemotherapy as initial treatment for metastatic colorectal cancer. *N Engl J Med* 2009;**360**:1408–141.

(5) Grothey A, Sugrue MM, Purdie DM *et al.* Bevacizumab beyond first progression is associated with prolonged overall survival in metastatic colorectal cancer: results from a large observational cohort study (BRiTE). *J Clin Oncol* 2008;**26**(33):5326–5334.

Oxaliplatin

Oxaliplatin is a platinum-based cytotoxic drug that prevents DNA replication by the formation of DNA cross-links. In general it is given in combination with 5-FU and is not used as a single agent. Common toxicities include; cumulative sensory peripheral neuropathy, which is often dose limiting, and myelosuppression. Hair loss is unusual.

Irinotecan

Irinotecan inhibits topoisomerase I, an enzyme that is essential for DNA replication. It may given as a single agent or in combination with 5-FU. Common toxicities include; diarrhoea,

myelosuppression, acute cholinergic symptoms (sweating, stomach cramps and diarrhoea) and alopecia.

Other conventional cytototoxic agents

Raltitrexed inhibits the enzyme thymidylate synthase. Its use is largely limited to patients who are intolerant of 5-FU. Mitomycin C is an alkylating agent with activity in colorectal cancer. It is used in combination with 5-FU.

Targeted chemotherapeutics

Over recent years the focus of drug development has moved away from conventional cytotoxic agents towards the development of agents that selectively target the molecular pathways involved in cancer growth. Molecular targeted agents currently approved for use in advanced colorectal cancer are; cetuximab and panitumumab, monoclonal antibody agents that target the epidermal growth factor receptor (EGFR) and bevacizumab, a monoclonal antibody that targets vascular endothelial growth factor (VEGF). The targeted chemotherapy agents have distinct side effect profiles which differ from the conventional cytotoxic drugs. The targeted chemotherapeutics for advanced disease are summarised below and discussed in detail in the following chapter.

Bevacizumab

Bevacizumab is given in combination with conventional cytotoxic chemotherapy schedules and has been shown to provide a survival benefit in both the first- and second-line setting. The main toxicities are: hypertension, slow wound healing, bleeding, increased risk of thromboembolic events. There is also a risk of perforation of the GI tract which occurs in 1.5–2.5% of patients.

Cetuximab (Chimeric IgG1) and Panitumumab (Fully humanised IgG2)

Clinical studies have demonstrated that the activity of these agents is limited to patients whose tumours express the wild-type *KRAS*

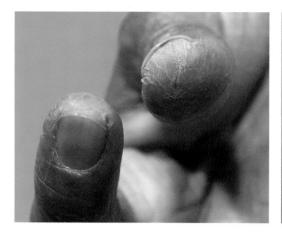
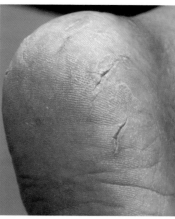

Figure 13.4 Palmar plantar erythema typically seen with 5-FU therapy. Dry cracked skin with fissuring is seen, involving the hands and feet. Treatment is with moisturising skin creams. A short interruption in 5-FU therapy may be necessary to allow recovery.

oncogene. Patients whose tumours harbour mutant *KRAS* do not gain any benefit from treatment. These findings have resulted in tumour *KRAS* testing gaining a clinical role in the selection of patients to receive these targeted therapies.

The initial clinical development of cetuximab was undertaken in the setting of chemorefractory disease (patients who had progressed on conventional cytotoxic chemotherapy), where early studies demonstrated that the combination of cetuximab and irinotecan could partial reverse resistance to irinotecan therapy. Subsequent trials evaluating the benefit of these agents when given in combination with conventional cytotoxic agents in the first- and second-line setting indicate that higher response rates and longer disease control can be achieved with this approach. The first-line use of cetuximab may be of particular benefit in patients with isolated liver metastasis allowing a higher proportion of patients to undergo attempt at curative resection. The main toxicities are: an acne-like skin rash (Figure 13.5), hypomagnesaemia and with cetuximab, infusion related hypersensitivity reactions.

Locoregional therapies for liver and lung metastasis

The liver is frequently the main site of disease involvement in patients with advanced disease and a variety of techniques have been developed to specifically target liver deposits. These include radiofrequency ablation (RFA), hepatic arterial infusion (HAI) chemotherapy and the infusion of radioactive microspheres (SIR-Spheres) into the hepatic artery. RFA may be used to treat liver or lung metastasis and is of particular use in patients considered high operative risk for resection. RFA may also be used as an adjunct to the surgical resection of liver metastasis. Developments allowing the delivery of high precision stereotactic radiotherapy such as CyberKnife are likely to play an increasing role in the management of isolated metastatic disease. SIR-Spheres are not commonly used in routine practice but may have a role in the management of patients with liver only disease. Advances in systemic chemotherapy have largely obviated the role of HAI chemotherapy in the treatment of advanced colorectal cancer.

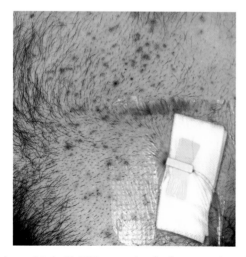
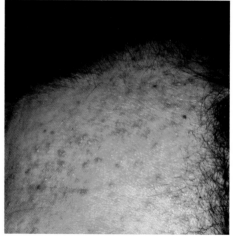

Figure 13.5 Skin rash associated with EGFR targeted antibodies. A pustular rash is evident on the chest and forehead. A correlation between severity of skin rash and response to EGFR targeted therapy has been seen in clinical trials. This patient is receiving intravenous therapy via an implanted venous access port. The access needle is visible on the chest wall.

Personalised therapy

The identification and evaluation of clinical biomarkers predictive of treatment response and/or toxicity is an emerging area of practice. Predictive biomarkers will play an increasing role in defining the use of both conventional cytotoxic agents and molecular targeted therapies in individual patients. The potential benefits include: lower toxicities, improved cost effectiveness and improved disease control. *KRAS* mutational testing is the only molecular marker currently in routine practice. Other molecular markers under evaluation include: gene mutations (i.e. BRAF, PIK3CA, PTEN), gene copy number variation (i.e. EGFR), gene polymorphisms and altered gene expression.

Symptomatic measures

Symptomatic and supportive care measures play an important role in the management of patients with advanced colorectal cancer. Symptoms may arise from either the disease itself or resulting from treatment received. Palliative care specialists in the hospital and community together with primary care services can help ensure that patients achieve optimal symptom control throughout the course of their disease. In certain scenarios interventional procedures can be beneficial. The use of self-expanding enteric stents in patients with obstructing primary tumours can allow the alleviation of obstructive symptoms without the need for surgical intervention. Radiotherapy may also be helpful in controlling symptoms arising from isolated sites of disease. As well as the physical symptoms of disease, patients also have to cope with the emotional impact of a cancer diagnosis. The provision of psychological support for patients and their families is an important aspect of care (Chapter 15).

Further reading

Guidance on Cancer Services: Improving Outcomes in Colorectal Cancers. Manual Update. National Institute for Clinical Excellence 2004. Available at http://www.nice.org.uk/guidance/CSGCC#documents [accessed 10 April 2011]. Refer to the NICE website http://www.nice.org.uk for current guidelines.

Leonard GD, Brenner B, Kemeny NE. Neoadjuvant chemotherapy before liver resection for patients with unresectable liver metastases from colorectal carcinoma. *J Clin Oncol* 2005;**23**(9):2038–2048.

Schilsky RL. Personalized medicine in oncology: the future is now. *Nature Reviews Drug Discovery*. May 2010;**9**:363–366.

CHAPTER 14

Innovative Treatment for Colorectal Cancer

Joanne L. Brady[1] *and David Kerr*[2]

[1]Department of Oncology, Churchill Hospital, Oxford, UK
[2]University of Oxford, Oxford, UK

OVERVIEW

- Despite improvements in surgery, chemotherapy and radiotherapy the overall survival for patients with metastatic colorectal cancer are still low. Improvements in understanding tumour biology has led to the development of targeted therapies

- Drugs which target the angiogenesis pathway have shown a survival advantage in patients with metastatic colorectal cancer

- Antibodies to the epidermal growth factor receptor show promise as single agents and in combination with chemotherapy

- The COX-2 pathway is known to have an important role in colorectal cancer development. However there are concerns regarding the safety of these drugs

- Gene therapy and immunotherapy show interesting results in early phase studies, but further investigation is awaited

Despite the many advances in conventional anti-cancer treatment over the last decade colorectal cancer remains the second highest cause of cancer deaths in the UK, with 32,000 new cases diagnosed and 13,000 deaths per year. Although the 5-year survival for early disease is now 80%, and there have been advances in adjuvant therapy which have significantly improved the outcome for patients with Stage III cancer, the median survival for those diagnosed with metastatic disease remains less than 24 months. Clearly new strategies to treat colorectal cancer are needed. A better understanding of the disease pathogenesis and tumour biology has led to the development of novel therapies with specific biological targets.

Angiogenesis and the VEGF pathway

In 1971 Judah Folkman first proposed that angiogenesis (the development of new blood vessels from the pre-existing vascular network) was essential for tumour growth and metastasis. Although angiogenesis is a complex multi-step pathway involving a large number of cytokines and cofactors, it has been established that the cytokine VEGF (vascular endothelial growth factor) and its receptor pathway are the key mediators. Normal cells undergo somatic mutations 'transforming' them into cancerous cells. These cells accumulate defects in regulatory circuits governing normal cellular proliferation. Such cancer cells proliferate to form small (1 to 2 mm) avascular tumours. In order to continue to grow, tumours secrete angiogenic factors, including VEGF, which stimulate the growth of new blood vessels. Access to a blood supply allows tumours to grow rapidly and to metastasise. Inhibition of angiogenesis may reverse this process, leading to regression of tumour vasculature and a correlative shrinking of the tumour. More than 50% of colon tumours express VEGF compared with minimal expression on normal colon tissue, and its expression has been shown to correlate with tumour stage and poor prognosis. It therefore presents an excellent target for a directed therapy (Figure 14.1).

Bevacizumab is a humanised monoclonal antibody that binds to and neutralises VEGF. It has been investigated in a number of clinical trials and has been shown to be well tolerated in the majority of patients with few side effects. As previously mentioned in Chapter 13, bevacizumab significantly improved overall survival when combined with irinotecan, 5FU and leucovorin (control group 15.6 months vs 20.3 months in the bevacizumab group (p < 0.001)) (Table 14.1). The side effects associated with bevacizumab are hypertension (which can be readily managed with anti-hypertensives), problems with wound healing and a small number of cases of bowel perforation and gastro-intestinal bleeding. Unfortunately this modest improvement in outcome comes at a high financial cost and bevacizumab has not been approved by NICE for this reason (December 2010). Its use in adjuvant therapy needs further thought (Chapter 12).

Other anti-VEGF agents are also currently in development, and of particular interest are small molecules, which have been specifically designed to inhibit the VEGF receptor. These have the advantage of being oral rather than intravenous (IV) preparations. Two large phase three studies have been carried out combining vatalanib (also called PTK/ZK) with chemotherapy; unfortunately there was no evidence of an overall survival benefit compared to controls who received chemotherapy alone (disease free survival was significantly increased in patients who were receiving valatanib plus chemotherapy as second line treatment for metastatic colorectal cancer). This lack of efficacy may be explained by the fact that the half-life of vatalanib is less than 5 hours. Taking this drug once a day, as in the study, therefore results only in intermittent inhibition

ABC of Colorectal Cancer, Second Edition.
Edited by Annie Young, Richard Hobbs and David Kerr.
© 2011 Blackwell Publishing Ltd. Published 2011 by Blackwell Publishing Ltd.

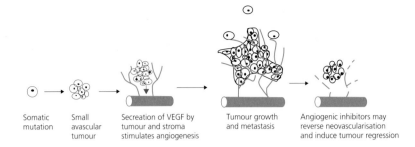

Figure 14.1 Angiogenesis as a target for anti cancer therapy.

Table 14.1 Results of phase 3 trial comparing IFL to IFL and bevacizumab (from Hurwitz *et al.*).

	IFL/Placebo	IFL/Bevacizumab	p Value
Median survival (mo)	15.6	20.3	<0.001
Progression-free survival (mo)	6.24	10.6	<0.001
Overall response rates	34.7%	44.9%	0.004
Duration of response (mo)	7.1	10.4	0.001

of the VEGF receptor. Future studies with this drug are likely to incorporate twice daily dosing.

Other novel agents targeting the VEGF signalling pathway also currently being investigated in combination with chemotherapy are AZD2171 (cedinarib) and sunitinib. Aflibercept, a humanised soluble VEGF receptor protein designed to act as a 'VEGF trap' is being tested in combination with 5-FU and irinotecan in second-line treatment of metastatic CRC.

Inhibitors of the epidermal growth factor receptor

The epidermal growth factor receptor (EGFR, also known as HER-1) is a cell-surface receptor which binds to various ligands and cytokines leading to cell division via the tyrosine kinase cascade EGFR, is over-expressed by 25–77% of colorectal cancers and is associated with a poor prognosis. The K-RAS protein is a key component of the EGFR pathway (Figure 14.2). Approximately 35% of colorectal cancers express an abnormal mutated form of K-RAS

which results in the pathway being permanently 'switched-on' leading to increased tumour cell proliferation, migration, angiogenesis and decreased apoptosis (programmed cell death) (Figure 14.2).

Cetuximab (Erbitux®) is a chimeric monoclonal antibody which binds to the EGFR preventing ligand-binding and receptor activation. This has been shown to have response rates in the region of 8–10% when given as a single agent in patients with irinotecan refractory CRC. When given in combination with irinotecan to patients with EGFR- expressing tumours who had irinotecan refractory disease the response rates are improved to 23% vs 11% with cetuximab alone. There was no evidence of a survival benefit due to crossover between the two arms of the study.

A study in Canadian and Australian patients with metastatic colorectal cancer showed a survival advantage in those treated with cetuximab compared to those treated with best supportive care, and on further analysis this was shown to be confined to those patients expressing the wild-type K-RAS protein. In a large multi-centre phase III study, response rates to treatment with cetuximab in combination with chemotherapy were significantly higher than those for chemotherapy alone (47% vs 39%), but more significantly this improvement was shown only in those patients who expressed wild-type K-RAS (RR 59% in this group). Cetuximab was of no clinical benefit in patients expressing the mutated K-RAS protein.

Panitumumab (Vectibix®) is a fully humanised monoclonal antibody which also targets the EGFR pathway. Although no formal comparisons between cetuximab and panitumumab have been made, it appears to be similar to cetuximab in mode of action and

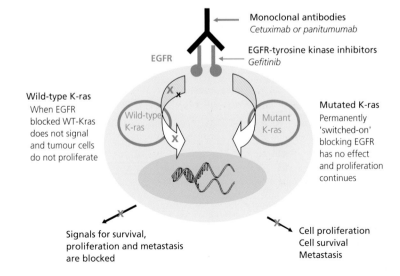

Figure 14.2 Anti EGFR therapy and K-RAS mutations.

single agent efficacy. Its beneficial effects are confined to colorectal cancer patients with wild-type K-RAS.

As panitumumab is a fully humanised antibody, the incidence of hypersensitivity with it is thought to be lower than with cetuximab, and this has been borne out in clinical trials.

Another agent targeting the EGFR pathway is the small molecule gefitinib (Iressa®), which is taken orally. This seems to be ineffective as a single agent but has been shown to have some promising activity when given in combination with 5-FU based drugs and oxaliplatin (with partial response rates of 75%) in patients with metastatic colorectal cancer.

EGFR-inhibitors appear to be very well tolerated with the only major side effects being allergic reactions, diarrhoea and an acneiform rash (Figure 14.3). The severity of the rash seems to correlate with the anti-tumour effect of the drug and a study was carried out wherein patients receiving cetuximab for metastatic colorectal cancer had the cetuximab dose increased until a rash developed. The response rate in this group was 30% vs 13% in those who had continued on the standard dose.

Anti-tumour vaccines

There has been increasing interest in exploiting the immune system to target cancer cells. There is evidence that certain cancers can be destroyed by tumour specific cell-mediated response, usually involving CD8 (cytotoxic) T-lymphocytes (Figure 14.4). In colorectal cancer the presence of a lymphocytic infiltrate at the primary site is known to correlate with late metastases and prolonged survival.

Immunotherapy using classic vaccination depends upon identifying a specific antigen on the surface of cancer cells (both primary

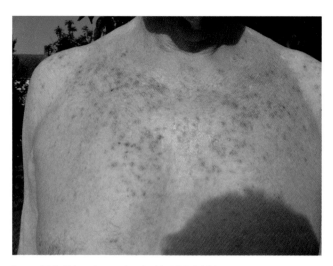

Figure 14.3 Skin rash associated with EGFR inhibitors.

and metastases), which is absent from normal tissue. Colorectal cancer cells do not usually elicit an immune response in the patient, because they are self-antigens and so have acquired 'tolerance', or because they lack co-stimulatory molecules such as the Major Histocompatability Complex (MHC). There are many different types of antigen that have been suggested as possible candidates for anti-cancer vaccines (see Table 14.2).

Tumour-derived whole cell vaccination

Rather than using an isolated antigen, whole cells derived from the patients' tumour have been used in trials, in combination

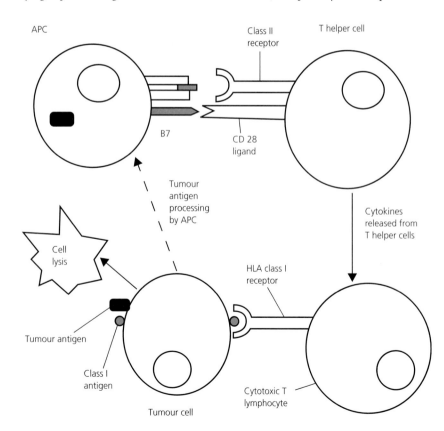

Figure 14.4 Cell-mediated immunity against tumours. Tumour antigens are taken up and processed by antigen presenting cells (APC), and presented to class II receptors on T-helper cells. An effective response requires the interaction between co-stimulatory signal, B7 and CD28 ligand, causing T-helper cell activation. As a consequence, cytokines (e.g. IL-2) are secreted from helper cells to activate tumour-specific cytotoxic lymphocytes to recognise tumour cells via class I receptors, and kill tumour cells.

Table 14.2 Biological targets for novel therapies.

Antigen type	Example
Heat shock protein	Cellular protein
Microenvironmental factors	VEGF, MMPs
Growth factor receptors	EGFR, Her-2
Mutated proteins	Ras, p53
Carbohydrate antigens	MUC-1
Glycoprotein antigens	CEA, 5T4

with BCG as an immunomodulatory adjuvant. These vaccines presumably contain a wide spectrum of tumour antigens and also have the advantage of being 'tailored' to the individual as biopsies of their own tumour are used as the basis of the vaccine. When trialled in the adjuvant setting there was some evidence of an immune response following vaccination, and in one study there was evidence of prolonged survival in a subset of early stage patients. However these trials did not include adjuvant chemotherapy, now considered the standard of care, and this approach has not entered widespread clinical use.

Virally encoded vaccines

This is a technique whereby a gene of interest is inserted into the genome of a viral vector that is injected as a vaccine with the aim of infecting host cells. This causes production of the protein of interest which is then presented to the immune system via the MHC by the patient's own antigen presenting cells. CEA (carcinoembryonic antigen) is a foetal protein expressed by the majority of colorectal cancers and it has been used as a target gene in trials using vaccinia virus. Although specific anti-CEA T cell immune responses were identified, and the vaccines were well tolerated, no tumour responses were seen.

5T4 is a glycoprotein expressed by more than 85% of colon cancers. Expression by normal gut cells is minimal. A vaccine has been developed to the 5T4 antigen (Trovax®), which in early phase studies has been shown to be safe and to produce an anti-5T4 immune response. When given in combination with chemotherapy the overall response rate was 60% vs 40% response rates to chemotherapy alone in historical controls. Further work is being carried out with this vaccine in the adjuvant setting.

Matrix metalloproteinase inhibitors

The matrix metalloproteinases (MMPs) are a family of 24 enzymes which degrade the extra-cellular matrix and are involved in the early stages of cancer cell invasion and metastasis. They have been shown to be over-expressed in many tumour types and are usually associated with a worse prognosis. Inhibitors of MMPs (e.g. marimastat, prinostat) have been developed, and one study in patients with CRC showed a dose-dependent reduction in CEA when treated with marimastat, but no obvious clinical benefit. It is thought the different MMPs have overlapping substrate specificity and the drugs inhibit only some of the isoenzymes, and therefore new generations of MMP inhibitors have wider specificities than their predecessors.

Cyclooxygenase 2 inhibitors

Cyclooxygenase 2 (COX2) is an intracellular enzyme that converts arachidonic acid into prostaglandins. High levels of COX2 and prostaglandin E2 are commonly found in colon tumour cells and there is laboratory evidence suggesting that the COX-2 pathway plays an important role in colorectal carcinogenesis during the transition from adenoma to carcinoma and subsequently during invasion and metastasis. Epidemiologic studies have indicated that the incidence of colorectal cancer is reduced by 30–70% in patients taking NSAIDS. A large randomised UK phase III study was therefore initiated in patients who had undergone potentially curative surgery for colorectal cancer to determine the role of rofecoxib (Vioxx®) in preventing tumour recurrence. Follow-up of the trial patients showed a moderate increase in serious cardiovascular events in patients on the treatment arm (1% for rofecoxib vs 0.5% for placebo) after rofecoxib was withdrawn from the market. The study (with only around a third of the target number of patients enrolled), was a negative one, showing no significant differences in outcomes with respect to overall, disease-free, or recurrence-free survival. The results of a similar large US study are awaited.

Gene therapy

Gene therapy is the transfer of genetic material via a vector into a patient's cells with the aim of directly or indirectly causing the demise of the cancerous cells.

One approach is gene-directed enzyme pro-drug therapy (GDEPT) where the gene for an enzyme, which can convert a pro-drug into an active metabolite, is transferred via a viral vector into tumour cells. This is a way of targeting tumour cells to avoid systemic side effects of chemotherapy (Figure 14.5). The major obstacle with this approach is the limited gene transfer efficiency with the currently available vectors, and therefore there is increasing interest in developing replication-proficient viruses

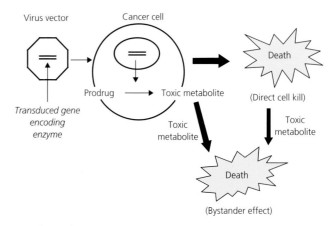

Figure 14.5 Virus directed enzyme pro-drug therapy. The gene encoding the enzyme to convert non-toxic pro-drug into toxic metabolite is inserted into cancer cell by a viral vector. The toxic metabolite can kill adjacent uninfected cancer cells via cell-to-cell contact or released from dead cell, i.e. bystander effect.

which can selectively infect and destroy cancer cells. The whole field has been somewhat held back by the test and technical barriers of manufacturing sufficient quantities of virus for even phase I/II trials, and investment needs to be made in biomanufacturing to create a sufficiently stable base from which to proceed to more definitive clinical development pathways.

Further reading

Cunningham D, Humblet Y, Siena S. Cetuximab monotherapy and cetuximab plus irinotecan in irinotecan-refractory metastatic colorectal cancer. *N Engl J Med* 2004;**351**:337–345.

Hurwitz H, Fehrenbacher L, Novotny W. Bevacizumab plus irinotecan, fluorouracil, and leucovorin for metastatic colorectal cancer. *N Engl J Med* 2004;**350**:2335–2342.

Kerr DJ, Dunn JA, Langman MJ. Rofecoxib and cardiovascular adverse events in adjuvant treatment of colorectal cancer. *N Engl J Med*;**357**:360–369.

National Institute for Health and Clinical Excellence. Bevacizumab and cetuximab for the treatment of metastatic colorectal cancer. Technology appraisal guidance 118. 2007.

Palmer D, Chen M-J, Kerr DJ. Gene therapy for colorectal cancer. *British Medical Bulletin* 2002;**64**:201–225

Van Cutsem E, Köhne C-H, Hitre E, *et al.* Cetuximab and chemotherapy as initial treatment for metastatic colorectal cancer. *N Engl J Med* 2009;**360**:1408–1417.

CHAPTER 15

Supportive Care for Patients with Colorectal Cancer

Pauline McCulloch[1] and Annie Young[2]

[1]Community Palliaitve Care CNS, London, UK
[2]Warwick Medical School, University of Warwick, Coventry, UK

OVERVIEW

- Healthcare professionals as part of a multidisciplinary team should address the patient and carer's supportive needs, best coordinated by a 'keyworker'. The colorectal cancer nurse specialist is often well placed to manage the supportive care pathway

- An holistic assessment of patient needs allows individualised care planning

- The key to effective pathway management is good communication between the multidisciplinary team and the patient and carer

- Patients with colorectal cancer who require stoma formation by and large experience more problems than those who do not; the support and advice of a stoma nurse specialist is widely recognised to be of great value

- There are novel technologies for monitoring the side effects of chemotherapy for colorectal cancer patients. International guidelines should be used for the management of side effects

Introduction

Kevin Bond's perspective of living with colorectal cancer [CRC] (Chapter 1) forms a fascinating description of the emotional impact of the disease on both the patient and family and offers counsel to all healthcare clinicians and managers on running a first-rate individualised service. As Kevin eloquently portrays, following a diagnosis of CRC, people undergo a period of emotional trauma as a result of their interpretation of the impact of the news they have just received. This trauma will be influenced by many factors such as:

- Previous life experiences, including any mental health issues.
- Previous experience of cancer either themselves or someone close.
- Their understanding of the diagnosis, prognosis and how it will impact on them and their loved ones.

ABC of Colorectal Cancer, Second Edition.
Edited by Annie Young, Richard Hobbs and David Kerr.
© 2011 Blackwell Publishing Ltd. Published 2011 by Blackwell Publishing Ltd.

- How the news was delivered about the diagnosis, that is the skills of the healthcare professional involved.
- The individual's social and supportive network that they can access for emotional and practical support.
- The availability of supportive healthcare professionals who can address the individuals information and supportive needs, that is access to a key worker.

Holistic patient assessment

It is important that all professionals in the multidisciplinary team (MDT), are able to recognise the factors above and identify and care for colorectal cancer patients experiencing emotional upset at different stages of their pathway (see Table 15.1 and Box 15.1), in addition to managing their specific area of expertise, such as colorectal surgery, stoma care, chemotherapy and so on. A comprehensive or 'holistic' baseline assessment is crucial in determining the optimal care interventions, be they psychological or the type of chemotherapy treatment best suited to the patient. This assessment will aid the MDT (e.g. using the decision support networks in Chapter 6), along with the patient, to map out a 'treatment' plan – Kevin's 'plan of action'. The assessment should include the emotional, psychological, social, spiritual, and sexual concerns as well as the 'medical' needs of the patient, and aim to work towards a

Table 15.1 Patients' emotional responses to the diagnosis of colorectal cancer.

Time of diagnosis	Fear, questions, anger, worry Uncertainty re outcome of treatments
During treatment	Change in body image as a result of stoma formation, scars, weight loss/gain, insertion of lines for chemotherapy Sexuality issues, loss of libido, pain, discomfort Altered bowel function following surgery
Living with cancer	Uncertainly re future, worry about recurrence Long term issues following treatment Adjusting to loss Medicalisation of life
Recurrence	Fear, anger, sadness and loss of future Recommencing treatment

resolution as a result of exploring concerns and helping the patients and their carers to find ways of managing them.

The National Institute for Health and Clinical Excellence (NICE) *Supportive and Palliative Care Guidance* (2004) is a first-rate and still contemporary publication, which offers direction on the assessment and interventions that address the impact of cancer on people's daily lives including family relationships, patients' mood, ability to work and financial hardship. The 'Distress Thermometer' is becoming more widely used in the UK as a fairly swift and effective screening and assessment tool for identifying such a spectrum of patient needs (Figure 15.1).

Box 15.1 Emotional responses to a diagnosis of colorectal cancer

Uncertainty

Patients need to be made aware that this is a normal response and then be given some mechanisms of managing this, part of which may be the contact details of their 'keyworker' or 'first point of contact' person, to seek advice from.

Sadness and depression

Sadness and sorrow can fluctuate throughout the patients' cancer pathway. Patients may manage these feelings by talking to family and friends, seeking help from a therapist, contacting patient help lines or support groups, talking to healthcare professionals or writing down their perceptions. However a few patients who experience mild and/or clinical depression following the diagnosis may be referred to a psychologist or psychiatrist with experience in working with people with cancer. Cognitive therapies, self-help and anti-depressants may be helpful for such patients.

Sexuality issues

The treatment that patients undergo for their CRC may negatively impact on their sexual desire and function. Male patients may experience loss of erectile ability after pelvic surgery or radiotherapy, this may be temporary or permanent, and it can also be unrelated to the surgery and may be a psychological response to the diagnosis. Female patients may experience loss of sensation, vaginal dryness due to surgical intervention or pelvic radiotherapy. It is beneficial for patients with sexuality concerns to be referred to a trained psychosexual counsellor for specialist assessment and therapy.

Communication

The golden key to the best possible care pathway is excellent communication between the healthcare team and, in turn, between the patient, carer and team, to facilitate exploration, consensus and coordination of care with dignity, respect and honesty, thus establishing trust. Health professionals have found advanced communications skills training useful in improving practice. Individual healthcare professionals are also aware of their limitations, and know when to refer onto a more appropriate person for specific patient or carer needs. Examples of key skills for communication are given in Box 15.2.

Box 15.2 Key skills for communication

Reflection: it's similar to being a mirror to what you've heard or understood in the verbal and non-verbal communication. It demonstrates that you are listening and hearing what is being said.

Paraphrasing: this is where the listener summarises what has been said to them, trying to help identify the key issues. It is also useful if there has been a lot of information to summarise it and then ask the person to identify what is important to them to explore more fully.

Active listening: this is listening to, hearing and understanding what is being communicated verbally and non-verbally. Using this skill encourages the listener to focus on the communication process.

Questioning: the use of open questions, encourages more complete answers. The use of such questions as 'how do you feel about . . . ' will give the person an opportunity to provide a more detailed answer.

Open questions usually start with how, what, why. Using closed questions is generally to obtain demographic, biographic or yes/no replies.

Nurses facilitating self-responsibility

The role of the colorectal nurse specialist is vital in providing information and support. Nurse-led follow up clinics provide continuity of care and information tailored to individual need (Chapter 16). Nurses, in particular, have an important role to play in ensuring that patients' perspectives and priorities for self-care are listened to and acted upon in order to help them achieve their desired level of involvement in self-care. Chemotherapy specialist nurses play a critical role in the detection and management of adverse effects resulting from chemotherapy regimens for CRC which are described in Chapters 12 and 13.

Management of side effects of chemotherapy for colorectal cancer

Chemotherapy

Standard chemotherapy regimens for CRC bring with them side effects of abdominal cramping and diarrhoea, nausea and vomiting, skin and hypersensitivity reactions, fatigue, stomatitis, neutropenia and thrombocytopenia, and alopecia (summarised in Table 15.2). The rigorous chemotherapy regimens often present patients with multiple obstacles in the activities of daily living, significantly impacting their quality of life. Educating patients about adverse treatment effects empowers them to manage their symptoms and enables them to alleviate serious or life-threatening treatment complications. General principles for the management of such side effects are outlined in Table 15.3. Personalised therapy may address each patient's potential therapeutic response and toxicity to specific chemotherapy agents, for example overexpression of thymidylate synthase may predict an inherent resistance to 5-FU; low expression of thymidine phosphorylase is associated with tumour response and survival; patients with dihydropyrimidine

Name: _____ Hospital number : _____ I am : ☐ The patient ☐ Relative / carer

1. Please circle the number (0-10) that best describes how much distress in general you have been experiencing over the past week, including today.

HIGH
DISTRESS

THERMOMETER

10
9
8
7
6
5
4
3
2
1
0

NO DISTRESS

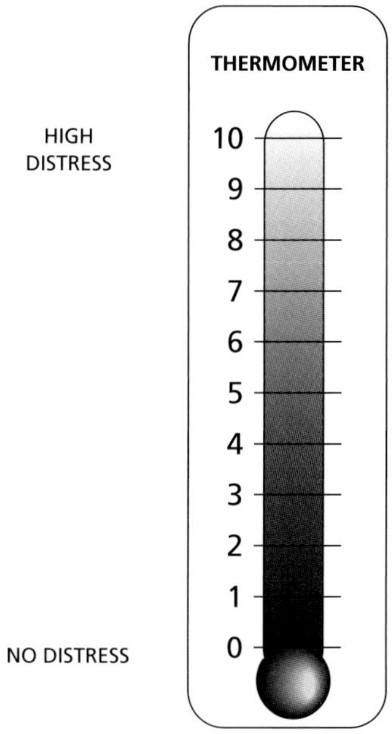

Distress Thermometer & Problem Checklist:
3 Counties Cancer Network amendment, 2006

2. If any of the following has been a problem for you over the past week, including today, please tick the box next to it. Leave it blank if it does not apply to you.

Practical Problems
☐ Child care
☐ Housing
☐ Finances
☐ Transport
☐ Work/school

Family Problems
☐ Dealing with children
☐ Dealing with partner

Emotional Problems
☐ Depression
☐ Fears
☐ Nervousness
☐ Sadness
☐ Worry
☐ Anger

Spiritual/religious Concerns
☐ Loss of faith
☐ Relating to God
☐ Loss of meaning or purpose of life

Communication Problems
☐ Amount of information
☐ Quality / clarity of information
☐ Communicating with staff

Physical Problems
☐ Appearance
☐ Bathing/dressing
☐ Breathing
☐ Changes in urination
☐ Constipation / Diarrhoea
☐ Concentration / Memory
☐ Eating
☐ Fatigue
☐ Feeling swollen / bloated
☐ Fevers / Hot flushes
☐ Getting around
☐ Indigestion
☐ Mouth sores
☐ Nausea and or Vomiting
☐ Nose dry/congested
☐ Pain
☐ Sexual
☐ Skin dry/itchy
☐ Sleep
☐ Tingling in hands/feet
☐ Metallic taste in mouth

Other _____

_____

3.FINALLY, out of the items you have ticked, please <u>underline</u> those that cause you the most concern (up to 4 items)

┌─────────────────────────────┐
│   │
│   │
│   Patient   │
│   details   │
│   │
│   │
└─────────────────────────────┘

To be completed by staff	
Signed by staff member:	Today's Date:
Diagnosis:	

Key concerns	Brief description of problem	Who is already helping?	Plan of action
1.			
2.			
3.			
4.			

Figure 15.1 Distress thermometer. Source: Jacobsen PB, Donovan KA, Trask PC, Heishman SB, Zabora J, Baker F, Holland JC. Screening for psychologic distress in ambulatory cancer patients *Cancer*, 2005;**103**(7):1494–502.

Table 15.2 Side effects of chemotherapy used to treat colorectal cancer.

System	Cytotoxic Agents				Targeted Therapies	
	5-FU/LV	Irinotecan	Oxaliplatin	Capecitabine	Bevacizumab (metastatic setting only)	Cetuximab
Bone marrow	Neutropenia	Neutropenia	Neutropenia	Neutropenia		
Gastro-intestinal	Mucositis Diarrhoea	Nausea and Vomiting Diarrhoea	Nausea and Vomiting Diarrhoea	Mucositis Nausea and Vomiting Diarrhoea	Gastrointestinal perforation	
Neurological			Acute self-limiting Chronic, cumulative			
Cardio-vascular					Hypertension Thrombosis Bleeding CHF	
Dermato-logical	Hand-foot syndrome Hyper-pigmentation			Hand-foot syndrome Hyperpigmentation	Delayed wound healing	Rash Paronychia Xerosis Trichomegaly (increased growth of eyelashes and eyebrows)
Renal					Nephrotic syndrome/ Proteinuria	
Other		Alopecia	Hypersensitivity, can occur with initial or subsequent doses			Infusion reactions (monitor patient for 1 hour post-infusional – longer if serious previous reaction) Hypomagnesemia, Hypokalaemia and Hypocalcaemia (monitor for 8 weeks post last dose) Interstitial lung disease (rare)

CRC – colorectal cancer; CHF – congestive heart failure; 5-FU – 5-fluorouracil; LV – leucovorin.

Table 15.3 General principles for management of side effects of chemotherapy for colorectal cancer.

(Evidence-based management guidelines to be used in everyday practice)

- **A comprehensive assessment prior to initiation of chemotherapy to be undertaken**
- **Reduce dose or stop relevant drug(s) as indicated in guidelines**

Be aware and be on hand to immediately treat any hypersensitivity with oxaliplatin and cetuximab infusions

Side effect	Principle
Neutropenia	Assess patient for risk of neutropenia in pre-chemotherapy check; Use ASCO, NCCN or EORTC Guidelines on Prevention and Management of Neutropenic Sepsis/Cancer-Related Infections.
Diarrhoea	Patient instructions must stress starting loperamide at the first sign of diarrhoea (change in consistency or frequency of stools) and to begin with 4 mg (2 tablets), followed by 2 mg every 2 hours until they have had no bowel movement for 12 hours.
Mucositis	Assess for neutropenic sepsis; promote good oral hygiene and use analgesia and antifungals and/or antibiotics for overlying infection.
Nausea and vomiting (N&V)	Assess risk of types of N&V in pre-chemotherapy check. Optimal emetic control in the acute phase is essential to prevent nausea and vomiting in the delayed phase; prophylaxis is better than treatment. Always commence anti-emetics before chemotherapy and give oral doses at least 30 minutes before chemotherapy. Anti-emetic therapy should be administered regularly and reviewed with each cycle of chemotherapy; initiate anti-emetics at lowest level appropriate for chemotherapy prescribed
Neuropathy	Oxaliplatin – reduce doses for chronic chemotherapy-induced neuropathy and discontinue the drug for persistent grade 3 neuropathy. Safety measures include wearing gloves when outdoors in cold weather, using potholders when cooking, wearing shoes when outdoors in both cold and warm weather to avoid frostbite or burns and using assistive devices (e.g. handrails and/or bathmats) as required.
Palmar-Plantar Erythrodysesthesia (PPE)/Hand-Foot Syndrome	Patients' shoes should be removed to examine feet properly. Patients should be instructed to stop capecitabine immediately if they develop grade 2 PPE or have manifestations that interfere with ADL. Symptomatic management e.g. using emollients to decrease skin drying. Patients should be asked to examine their skin and promptly report PPE manifestations to their keyworker and to avoid increased pressure to hands and feet from exercise and avoid increased exposure to heat.
Cardiovascular	For patients receiving bevacizumab, monitor blood pressure, assess for bleeding and thrombosis and test urine for proteinurea routinely. Refer to specialist in area of concern.
Rash Paronychia	Cetuximab – local comfort measures (i.e. warm soaks or compresses) may partially relieve discomfort, moisturisers and emollients may relieve dry skin and topical steroids may diminish erythema. Treat any overlying infection with antibiotics.

ASCO – American Society of Clinical Oncology; NCCN – National Comprehensive Cancer Network; EORTC – European Organisation for Research and Treatment of Cancer.

dehydrogenase deficiency may experience potentially fatal toxicity from 5-FU or severe stomatitis, diarrhoea, neutropenia and neurotoxicity with capecitabine.

New care pathway and technologies for monitoring the side effects of chemotherapy

We are currently testing and rolling out novel services for monitoring side effects of chemotherapy in patients with colorectal cancer who are receiving capecitabine. Patients are offered a specially programmed mobile phone (or they can use their own should they wish) to allow them to record how they feel, enter information on specific side effects and obtain advice about what steps to take to manage these side effects. In addition, the phone automatically alerts specialist chemotherapy nurses, who will contact the patient (where there are concerns) in a timely manner and according to the severity of the toxicity, to offer further support to reduce side effects and improve the patients' wellbeing. The dose intensity of capecitabine

is also being optimised automatically using the same mobile phone technology for patients with CRC, in a research setting.

Rehabilitation

In 2009, an outstanding rehabilitation pathway for patients with CRC was published by allied health professional specialists with the Cancer Action Team in England, in order to maximise the individuals' potential in many areas (e.g. nutrition and exercise and physical wellbeing) at every point in the pathway – 'diagnosis and care planning' to 'end of life'. Putting this pathway into daily practice for patients with CRC is the challenge for the MDT.

Stoma care

Adapting to life with a stoma involves a number of physical and psychological challenges, and the relationship formed between a patient and a stoma nurse specialist is vital to a smooth transition. Stoma care patients require support and guidance on issues such as stoma management and personal nutrition in order to improve the patient's social and personal confidence levels. The stoma nurse specialist also plays a key role in the rehabilitation process, by providing information and education, as well as encouragement and counselling for patients and their carers, all of whom have a diverse range of fears, needs and aspirations.

Financial issues

The diagnosis and ongoing treatment for CRC can be lengthy, resulting in the loss of employment and subsequent loss or reduction of income, adding an extra burden of worry. Therefore healthcare professionals need to address the question of financial issues with patients, and identify where relevant the need for benefits advice. If any financial need is identified, the patient and their carer should be referred to their local benefits officer, cancer information centre, Citizens Advice Bureau, or social worker to ensure they get support to alleviate any anxiety caused by such worries.

Palliative care

The main priorities in palliative care of patients with CRC include the management of pain, jaundice, ascites, constipation and nausea. The importance of attempting to correct these symptoms cannot be overstated; great distress may be caused by constipation or nausea as by pain. Full explanations of signs such as jaundice are likely to be reassuring. Moreover, the advent of specialist home care teams (with access to specialist equipment – such as bed aids to preserve pressure areas or syringe drivers for pain control) and skilled counsellors for patients and their families, enables virtually all patients who wish it to have specialist palliative care at home.

Conclusion

A diagnosis of colorectal cancer and its subsequent treatment can have a devastating impact on the quality of a person's life, as well as on the lives of their carers. Patients face new fears and uncertainties and may have to undergo unpleasant and debilitating treatments outlined in the previous chapters. They and their carers need access to support from the specialist CRC MDT from the time that cancer is first suspected, through all stages of treatment to recovery or, in some cases, to death and for the carers, into bereavement.

Further reading

Hallquist Viale P and Sommers R. Nursing care of patients receiving chemotherapy for metastatic colorectal cancer: implications of the treatment continuum concept. *Seminars in Oncology Nursing* 2007;**23**(1): 22–35.

Larouche S, and Edgar L. The measure of distress: A practical thermometer for outpatient screening. *Oncology Exchange* 2004;**3**(3):34–39.

National Cancer Rehabilitation Colorectal Care Pathways: http://www.cancer.nhs.uk/rehabilitation/documents/pathways/care_pathways/NCAT_Rehab_Colorectal.pdf [accessed 10 April 2011].

NICE Supportive and Palliative Care Guidance (2004) http://guidance.nice.org.uk/CSGSP/Guidance/pdf/English [accessed 10 April 2011].

Weaver A, Young AM, Rowntree J, Townsend N, Pearson S, Smith J, Gibson O, Cobern W, Larsen M, Tarassenko L. Application of mobile phone technology for managing chemotherapy-associated side-effects. *Ann Oncol.* 2007;**18**(11):1887–1892.

CHAPTER 16

Follow-up

John Primrose

Southampton General Hospital, Southampton, UK

OVERVIEW

- The aim of follow-up is to detect recurrence/metastatic/ metachronous disease at an earlier stage when it might improve outcome

- The area most likely to fulfil the above aims are the detection of metachronous polyps and cancer and operable liver and perhaps lung metastases

- Controversy exists as to which, if any, type of follow-up is best but a number of clinical trials are in progress

- It is of great importance that the patient is fully staged with CT chest abdomen and pelvis, 'clean' colon and normal CEA before a follow-up protocol is instituted

- At present a combination of a single CT and regular CEA measurements plus colonic imaging at 5 years is a reasonable strategy

- New prognostic markers are likely to be available soon to allow follow-up to be individualised

---

Introduction

It is relatively commonplace for clinicians to follow-up patients who have had resections for colorectal cancer, even though the evidence base to support this is far from robust. The aim of follow-up should be to detect recurrent disease at a stage where better outcomes can be achieved than if the patient presented with symptoms. It may be also be employed to detect and treat metachronous polyps or cancer. Follow-up may provide some psychological reassurance for the patient, though this is difficult to quantify. It may also contribute to audit, although it is probably not the most efficient means of achieving this.

In healthcare systems where funding is by item of service, such as the USA, there is clearly is an incentive to undertake a follow-up schedule which involves performing procedures. In a national healthcare system such as the NHS this incentive does not exist, indeed it adds to cost. Possibly for this reason there is an increasing move to nurse led follow-up based on a protocol or follow-up in primary care in the UK.

ABC of Colorectal Cancer, Second Edition.
Edited by Annie Young, Richard Hobbs and David Kerr.
© 2011 Blackwell Publishing Ltd. Published 2011 by Blackwell Publishing Ltd.

Sites of recurrence and treatment options

As with most malignancies, colorectal cancer may recur in a large number of sites. However, only a few are sufficiently common to be of major interest in terms of the follow-up schedule. Recurrent disease can be treated by a number of modalities, including surgery, radiotherapy and chemotherapy (Chapters 11, 10 and 13 respectively). At present only surgery is curative apart from in exceptional circumstances. Different sites and circumstance of recurrence may be more or less amenable to treatment. It also must be understood that the biology of the disease is overwhelmingly important in terms of outcome regardless of the type of treatment offered.

Liver metastases

A great deal of evidence is available to support the role of liver surgery in curing patients with recurrence (Figure 16.1). Indeed, if there is benefit from following up patients with colorectal cancer, it is most likely to be in detecting patients who might undergo liver resection.

It is self-evident that the liver metastasis must occur while the primary is still in situ. If metachronous liver metastasis appear it simply means that either the liver has not been sufficiently well examined to detect metastases at presentation or that at the time the disease was below the resolution of imaging techniques employed. It is evident now that with adequate staging of the patient preoperatively and the use of new generation scanners, particularly CT scans and sometimes MRI, that the number of patients with synchronous metastases detected is increased. Consequently fewer patients develop liver metastases later. This stage migration is critical when considering the cost effectiveness of follow-up schedules.

Lung metastases

Although the evidence base to support resection of lung metastases from colorectal cancer is less well developed than for liver, the results of resection are similar. Indeed a systematic review suggests in fact that the results may be somewhat better, but patient selection may play a part. There is no doubt that patients with resectable lung metastases do form a relatively small proportion of cases of colorectal cancer. However there may be sufficient incidences of curative resection to justify consideration of detection in a follow-up programme.

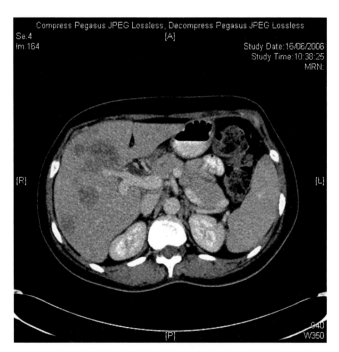

Compress Pegasus JPEG Lossless, Decompress Pegasus JPEG Lossless
Se:4   [A]
Im:164   Study Date:16/06/2006
                                Study Time:10:38:25
                                              MRN:
[R]   [L]
                                              [P]   C40
                                                     W350

Figure 16.1 MRI scan on the liver showing extensive but operable colorectal liver metastases. The patient is alive and well 7 years after liver resection.

Locoregional and peritoneal recurrence

Although incidences of cure are reported in patients who developed local or regional recurrence from colorectal cancer, this is uncommon. Most patients who develop such recurrence will die of disease. Although it may be treatable with cytotoxic chemotherapy or, in the pelvis, radiotherapy, there is no real evidence to support the contention that finding such disease before it becomes apparent symptomatically is of benefit. Hence follow-up directed towards detecting locoregional recurrence may not be justified at present.

Peritoneal metastasis carries a bad prognosis. Radical surgical approaches have been applied to peritoneal disease, similar to that which are employed for pseudomyxoma peritonei. In general terms although a subgroup may benefit there is little evidence to support cytoreductive surgery and intraperitoneal chemotherapy in this group. Therefore at present this approach probably does not have a place outside of clinical trials.

Surgical approaches have been employed for local recurrence from rectal cancer. However, if original treatment of the rectal cancer has been of good quality, including appropriate chemoradiotherapy and a good surgical technique, the results from a re-resection are not good. It would therefore be hard to justify follow-up to detect this disease at an asymptomatic stage.

Luminal recurrence and metachronous polyps and cancer

If the original surgical treatment has been adequate an actual luminal recurrence should be very rare. Luminal manifestation of locoregional recurrence certainly occurs but follow-up to detect this alone is not justified. By contrast, metachronous polyps and cancer are of considerable importance. Patients with colorectal cancer are predisposed to develop further polyps (Figure 16.2)

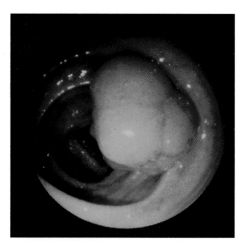

Figure 16.2 Colonoscopic follow-up of a patient with previous colorectal cancer showing metachronous polyp.

and ultimately metachronous cancer and there is therefore clear evidence to support surveillance of the colon in this setting (see the Association of Coloproctology and SIGN guidelines). It is firstly critical that synchronous polyps and cancer are excluded at the time of the original resection. This is something that can be overlooked as the presenting malignancy may preclude detailed examination of the remainder of the colon. This is particularly the case when the patient presents as an emergency. Therefore, before a follow-up strategy is implemented, the entire colon must be examined to determine whether there are any other polyps or missed synchronous cancers. Assuming this is done the evidence at present would support a further colonoscopy at around 5 years.

Other sites of recurrence

Bone, skin and brain metastases from colorectal cancer are all recognised. They reflect systemic disease and are not commonly curable. There is no suggestion a follow-up strategy might be devised to detect these.

Follow-up techniques

A number of techniques have been used to follow-up patients who had colorectal cancer with different levels of success.

Clinical follow-up with examination

In brief, there is no evidence to suggest that simple clinical follow-up with clinical examination has any place in the detection of treatable recurrent disease. It may serve to reassure a patient, falsely in many cases. It may aid data collection but at a significant cost in healthcare terms. It is, however, important to separate clinical review for follow-up from review of a clinically symptomatic patient. For instance, patients who have had rectal excisions often complain of a variety of symptoms which may need advice or treatment. This is not follow-up in the context of this article.

CT imaging

CT is currently the best form of follow-up imaging overall in patients who have had colorectal cancer. Whether CT should be employed and at what frequency is discussed below. Other imaging techniques all have deficiencies as outlined in Chapter 8.

Serum tumour marker measurements

Measurement of the most widely used and accepted tumour marker CEA (carcinoembryonic antigen) is simple to perform, inexpensive and has an acceptable specificity and sensitivity even in patients in whom an elevation could not be detected preoperatively. Systematic reviews and other studies suggest it to be of value in follow-up, and although to date there is no evidence base to suggest that in isolation, its use can save life. It does form part of the strategy in many follow-up trials considered in the various meta-analyses. Clinical interpretation is needed in using CEA measurements. Different values will sometimes be found between tests and higher levels tend to be found in smokers. What is important is the trend, and continually rising CEA measurement after measurement is highly indicative of recurrent disease. The tumour marker itself will give no clue at all as to the site of the recurrent disease. Its value is that it can trigger other investigations such as CT. However its simplicity, lack of invasiveness and the sensitivity make it an extremely promising part of any protocol follow-up.

Endoscopic imaging and virtual endoscopy

As detailed above, patients who have had colorectal cancer are predisposed to develop further polyps and cancer. For this reason there is very strong support for some form of endoscopic follow-up. At present colonoscopy is the investigation of choice as it can be therapeutic as well as diagnostic as polyps can be removed.

Colonoscopy is an invasive technique and therefore carries some risk. CT colonography is much less invasive but is associated with a radiation dose and in addition any polyps detected would then have to be removed by an endoscopic technique. However the CT colonography may in the future form part of a follow-up protocol in some patients.

Follow-up: the evidence

Systematic reviews and meta-analysis

A number of randomised trials have examined the utility of follow-up following potentially curative surgery for colorectal cancer. None of these trials are in themselves adequate. A multiplicity of problems are obvious. Commonly the trials are inadequately powered. There is huge diversity in the modalities employed and the intensity of follow-up is highly variable. None of them have used current standard of care imaging, nor have employed modern surgical or oncological techniques to deal with recurrent disease when found.

Four systematic reviews including a Cochrane review have considered all of the evidence from the randomised trials on follow-up. They have all essentially analysed the same papers and whilst three of the reviews conclude that there is a lack of evidence to support follow-up the fourth, using the same data set, suggests that there is. Therefore, controversy remains.

Of all the reviews, the Cochrane review is most rigorous. It showed there was overall survival benefit at 5 years for patients

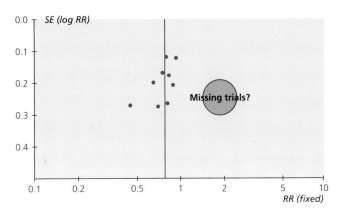

Figure 16.3 Funnel plot of studies reviewed in Cochrane Database Systematic Reviews (see reading list). The standard error of the risk ratio (related to the size of the trial) is plotted against the risk ratio. The asymmetrical appearance of the plot is typical of one in which smaller negative trials are missing as they are unreported. Produced by Ronald Koretz, California, (unpublished and used by permission).

undergoing more intensive follow-up with an odds ratio of 0.73 (95% confidence intervals 0.592-0.91). Interestingly it was hard to determine the cause of this apparent improvement in survival, as surgical treatment of recurrent disease did not seem to be a major contributing factor. All of this does raise the possibility of publication bias. The funnel plot (Figure 16.3) shows a very typical pattern suggesting that smaller negative trials may have been unpublished. Thus although follow-up using appropriate methodologies may well be useful in improving the outlook in patients treated for colorectal cancer, the evidence to date does not convincingly support this.

Ongoing trials

There are 3 trials currently ongoing addressing the issue of the utility of follow-up with very different designs. All of them essentially are examining the same group of patients; that is those with the curatively resected colorectal cancer in Duke's stages A-C (Stages I-III). The Italian Guilda Trial examines regular clinical review, CEA, colonoscopy, chest x-ray and liver ultrasound, compared to regular clinical review and CEA and infrequent colonoscopy and liver ultrasound. To date this trial has not reported benefit of the more intensive programme but it is noteworthy that all the patients have regular CEA performed.

The UK FACS trial examines regular CT imaging and CEA measurement compared to a single CT at 12 to 18 months postoperatively and no CEA in a 2x2 trial design. This trial has completed recruitment of 1,200 patients. Initial results (unpublished), and not by intervention group, show a low overall relapse rate. In those who relapse, a high instance of surgically incurable disease is noted. A possible interpretation of these findings is that the detailed staging of these patients prior to trial entry meant that many of the patients with metastatic disease were picked up at the time of the initial presentation or during adjuvant treatment.

The Scandinavian-based COLFOL study has the most intensive form of schedule studying regular CEA, CT/MRI and/or PET scanning at 6-monthly intervals for 2 years and again at 36 months, compared to CEA and CT/MRI of the liver at 12 and 36 months after surgery.

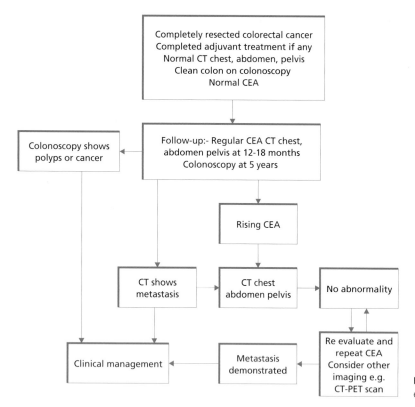

Figure 16.4 An algorithm for follow-up based on existing evidence.

Conclusions

In advance of the results of the modern trials being made available, it is possible to design a schedule for follow-up which is consistent with the current evidence base (Figure 16.4). This is also compatible with some of the existing published guidance.

First it is essential that the patient is adequately staged before they enter into a follow-up protocol. This means that they are free of metatastic disease on a CT scan that includes the chest, abdomen and pelvis. Next, they should have a 'clean colon' on appropriate imaging which might be colonoscopy or CT colonography. If this has not been performed prior to the operation, it should be undertaken before the patient goes into follow-up.

Lastly, the CEA should be found to be normal in the postoperative period. If the CEA is going to be used as part of the follow-up schedule, it is better that it is measured preoperatively, but in fact the evidence shows that even in the absence of this it retains value.

In terms of the follow-up methods, there is no evidence to support a clinical review once the patient is asymptomatic following the operation, and has no continuing complication being managed. However a means of rapidly reentering specialist care if needed is reassuring to a patient. This can be readily provided by a clinical nurse specialist or General Practitioner with an appropriate interest. A single postoperative CT around 12–18 months seems a reasonable option based on the evidence. Most recurrences in the liver will be evident by this stage. Lastly, bearing in mind its simplicity and lack of expense, 6-monthly CEA for several years might be reasonable.

Assuming follow-up is commenced, it is uncertain for how long it should be continued. Most recurrence will happen within 2 years and almost all by 5 years. There is, however, the occasional patient who will relapse later than 5 years, therefore continuing an annual CEA measurement until 10 years may not be inappropriate.

A colonoscopy, or if preferred a CT colonography, may be performed at around 5 years although some clinicians might prefer to do this earlier.

Lastly any follow-up protocol must be driven by the individual circumstances of the patient. There are many elderly patients who survive resection of the primary disease but would be disinclined to have any further treatment. Hence, follow-up in this particular situation is not indicated. By contrast, a younger patient with more aggressive disease might, for purposes of reassurance, warrant follow-up which is more intensive than that suggested.

It is likely that the issue of which patients require follow-up will come to the fore in the next few years. Biological factors in the tumours and host factors such as the immune response in the host are now being studied and are yielding important prognostic information. It is most likely that it will soon prove possible to identify a group of patients in whom recurrence is so unlikely that follow-up might be minimal. By contrast there will also be patients at very high risk in whom more intensive monitoring may be cost effective. These new prognostic methods will radically change the cost effectiveness of follow-up away from the blunt instrument it is at the moment.

Further reading

Association of Coloproctology of Great Britain and Ireland. *Guidelines for the Management of Colorectal Cancer*, 2007. Association of Coloproctology of Great Britain and Ireland. 3rd ed.

Jeffery M, Hickey BE, Hider PN. Follow-up strategies for patients treated for non-metastatic colorectal cancer. *Cochrane Database Syst Rev*, 2007: CD002200.

Mirnezami AH, Sagar PM. Surgery for recurrent rectal cancer: technical notes and management of complications. *Tech Coloproctol* 2010;**14**: 209–216.

Morris EJ, Forman D, Thomas JD, Quirke P, Taylor EF, *et al.* Surgical management and outcomes of colorectal cancer liver metastases. *Br J Surg* 2010;**97**:1110–1118.

Pages F, Galon J, Dieu-Nosjean MC, Tartour E, Sautes-Fridman C, *et al.* Immune infiltration in human tumors: a prognostic factor that should not be ignored. *Oncogene* 2010;**29**:1093–1102.

Primrose J, Treasure T, Fiorentino F. Lung metastasectomy in colorectal cancer: is this surgery effective in prolonging life? *Respirology* 2010;**15**:742–746.

Primrose JN. Surgery for colorectal liver metastases. *Br J Cancer* 2010;**102**:1313–1318.

Primrose JN, Fuller A, Rose P, Perera-Salazar R, Mellor J, Corkhill A, George S, Mant D. Follow-up after colorectal cancer surgery: Preliminary observational findings from the UK FACS trial. *J Clin Oncol* 2011;**29**:(suppl; abstr 3521).

Scottish Intercollegiate Guidelines Network. *Management of Colorectal Cancer: A National Clinical Guideline*, 2003. Edinburgh, Scottish Intercollegiate Guidelines Network.

Simmonds PC, Primrose JN, Colquitt JL, Garden OJ, Poston GJ, *et al.* Surgical resection of hepatic metastases from colorectal cancer: a systematic review of published studies. *Br J Cancer* 2006;**94**:982–999.

Tan E, Gouvas N, Nicholls RJ, Ziprin P, Xynos E, *et al.* Diagnostic precision of carcinoembryonic antigen in the detection of recurrence of colorectal cancer. *Surg Oncol* 2009;**18**:15–24.

Tejpar S, Bertagnolli M, Bosman F, Lenz HJ, Garraway L, *et al.* Prognostic and predictive biomarkers in resected colon cancer: current status and future perspectives for integrating genomics into biomarker discovery. *Oncologist* 2010;**15**:390–404.

Verwall VJ. Long-term results of cytoreduction and HIPEC followed by systemic chemotherapy. *Cancer J* 2009;**15**:212–215.

Index

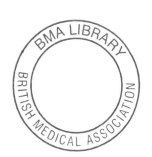

ABC of Interventional Cardiology

2ND EDITION

Ever D. Grech, Northern General Hospital, Sheffield

- Provides an easy to read, practical guide presenting the complex aspects of interventional cardiology in a clear and concise manner
- Explains the different interventions for coronary artery disease, ordered by clinical setting
- Covers the core knowledge on techniques and management, and highlights the evidence base.
- Illustrated in full colour throughout, with new images and graphics, it includes key guidelines, new drug treatments and devices, and further reading and resources in each chapter

DECEMBER 2010 | 9781405170673 | 120 PAGES | £24.99/US$38.95/€32.90/AU$49.95

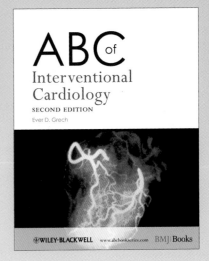

ABC of Learning and Teaching in Medicine, 2ND EDITION

Edited by Peter Cantillon & Diana Wood
National University of Ireland, Galway; University of Cambridge

- Emphasises the teacher's role as a facilitator of learning rather than a transmitter of knowledge
- Designed to be practical and accessible and support good teachers in becoming even better at what they do
- Seeks to explain how different aspects of learning and assessment work (the theory) as well as providing descriptions of educational approaches that work (the practice)
- Features core medical education topics such as course design, assessment, learning in groups, feedback, and the creation of learning materials
- Includes invaluable new chapters that address many of the challenges of medical education such as dealing with students in difficulty, the teaching of professionalism in clinical settings, and how to support the development of teachers

JULY 2010 | 9781405185974 | 96 PAGES | £22.99/US$33.95/€29.90/AU$47.95

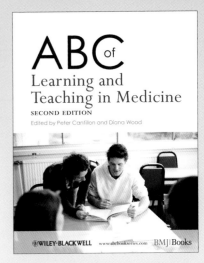

ABC of Clinical Leadership

Edited by Tim Swanwick & Judy McKimm, London Deanery; Unitec, New Zealand

- Written by clinical educators involved in running leadership programmes for doctors and other healthcare professionals
- Defines the scope of clinical leadership to emphasise its importance in the clinical context
- Develops and explores the key principles of leadership and management, and outlines the main leadership theories that have influenced health care practice
- Considers the challenges and skills in leading multi-disciplinary health care teams as well as the key factors involved in the leadership and management of change both at an individual and organisational level
- Considers a systematic approach to leading clinical services, strategic planning, and the management of people and resources
- Covers educational leadership, collaborative working and the importance of leading ethically and with integrity

DECEMBER 2010 | 9781405198172 | 88 PAGES | £19.99/US$30.95/€25.90/AU$39.95

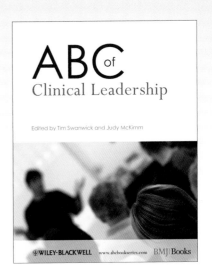

For more information on any of these books, please visit the ABC website at **www.abcbookseries.com**